Metadata

1st edition.

Table of Contents

Introduction

In this book, I have one premise: that making positive changes to your lifestyle can make you feel better, reduce your anxiety and increase your happiness.

Everybody has some degree of anxiety. If you are reading this, you probably feel that your level of anxiety is too high. Perhaps it is at a clinical level, known as *acute anxiety*, or perhaps not, but still has a significant effect on your life.

If so, you have probably felt this way for some time. For a few people, anxiety springs up on them after a change in life circumstances or traumatic event. For most people, however, anxiety has been there for years or decades.

If you have been living with anxiety for a prolonged period, you might think there is nothing you can do about it. This is not the case. There are treatments that can help, and there are changes you can make to your life to make you feel better.

These remedies do not have to be medication, and it does not have to be therapy. Making positive changes to your lifestyle, to be more "anxiety-friendly", can provide you with benefits that are even more powerful.

Who is this book aimed at?

This book is for anyone who feels that anxiety has a noticeable impact on their life. It is for those would like to better control their anxiety and be happier.

It is not aimed at anyone who is looking for a quick-fix cure for anxiety. Those do not exist, but even if they did, quick-fixes would be outside the scope of this book. This book is for people who are looking to make long-term changes in their life that result in lasting and positive improvements.

How is the book laid out?

In part one we will look at the importance of lifestyle and put it in context with anxiety. That means I will be explaining what anxiety is, and why we should focus on lifestyle to make improvements.

In part two, we will look at how we make changes. No matter what area of your life you are focusing on, there are some important guidelines for implementing changes, which you need to follow if you want to succeed.

In part three, we will look at the different lifestyle factors that can affect anxiety, and what changes and improvements you can make to each of them.

What exactly is lifestyle?

Lifestyle is a catch-all term for the way you live your life. This could include a lot of different factors, but in this book, I am going to look at these specific factors:

Exercise covers physical activity, going outside and enjoying nature.

Diet covers what you what, drink, and other things you may put in your body.

Sleep covers the quality and duration of your sleep, bedtime habits and routine.

Relaxation covers what you do to unwind, how you treat yourself and work life balance.

Personal growth covers personal development, learning new skills and keeping your brain active.

Relationships covers building your support network of family and friends.

Community covers interacting with the wider community, joining other social groups and making use of local peer support groups.

Between them, these seven broad topics cover the significant aspects of our lives that affect how we feel. The categories are not exclusive: some of them overlap in content.

What about mindfulness?

You may have heard that mindfulness is an effective technique for controlling anxiety, and that you should incorporate it into your schedule.

This is true. Mindfulness does seem to be effective for anxiety and there is lots of evidence to back this up1.

Mindfulness seems to be most effective when it is incorporated into your daily schedule2.

However, I will not be discussing mindfulness meditation in this book. There are lots of good books out there that already provide a comprehensive introduction to mindfulness meditation. My book, **Technical Anxiety**3, devotes a chapter to it.

Instead, in this book, I will look at how we can incorporate some mindfulness techniques into our everyday activities. For example how we can exercise, cook and enjoy life in a more mindful way.

There is no rush

There is no rush to get to the end of this book. In fact, I highly recommend that you deliberately do not rush to finish it. To get the most out of it, take it slow.

As anxiety sufferers it is easy to get caught up on the motorway of getting things done as fast as possible. We speed through every book, every exercise, every task, desperate to finish each and tick it off our to-do list without taking anything in.

That is the last thing we want to do here. To make lasting change, we need to take action. Having the knowledge is not enough. Reading the book will not make any changes to your life. It is through action, going out and doing things, that change will come.

---

1 Strauss C, Cavanagh K, Oliver A, Pettman D. Mindfulness-Based Interventions for People Diagnosed with a Current Episode of an Anxiety or Depressive Disorder: A Meta-Analysis of Randomised Controlled Trials. Laks J, ed. PLoS ONE. 2014;9(4):e96110. doi:10.1371/journal.pone.0096110.

2 Brown CA, Jones AK. Meditation experience predicts less negative appraisal of pain: electrophysiological evidence for the involvement of anticipatory neural responses. Pain. 2010 Sep;150(3):428-38. doi: 10.1016/j.pain.2010.04.017. Epub 2010 May 21. DOI: 10.1016/j.pain.2010.04.017

3 Chris Worfolk. Technical Anxiety: The complete guide to what is anxiety and what to do about it. ISBN: 978-1539424215

In that sense, this book will not help you directly. The book is more of a guide, a companion, to making the changes you want to make to improve your life. Simply reading the book cover to cover only puts you at the start of the journey, and not the end.

So slow down, and take your time.

How do you do this in practice? There are several ways. Perhaps you read a chapter at a time and only allow yourself to move on once you have done a set number of exercises.

Or perhaps you read it through from start to finish, then move your bookmark back to the start and work through it again, actually making the changes this time.

Case study

Alex was desperate to find a cure for her anxiety. It was all she could think about. She spent all her time reading as many books as possible, looking up information on the internet and trying to find as many ideas as possible until she had found the perfect one.

Every week she would find a new book on anxiety, order it and read it through as fast as she could. By the next week, she would have moved on to a new book and forgotten everything in the old one. The cycle went on and on.

In contrast, Amy decided to take it slowly. She picked up one book at a time and read one chapter per week. After reading the chapter, she would take the time to do all of the exercises that the book suggested.

It took her around 12 weeks to get through each book. However, with each one, she was able to make lasting changes to her lifestyle, including mindfulness meditations, more exercise and practising new thought patterns. After nine months she found she was thinking about her anxiety much less and was happier with her life.

Use of case studies

I use case studies regularly in this book. These are based on real-world examples and help illustrate each of the points I make. Do read the case studies.

In most cases, you will find the case study reinforces what you have just read, rather than tells you anything new. Therefore, you might be tempted to skip them. It is important not to do this.

First, reinforcing knowledge is important. Sometimes I may say the same thing repeatedly, and it may feel a little patronising. If you feel this way, I will apologise in advance. These feelings are normal, but it is important to stick with the book. Reinforcement is critical when it comes to tackling anxiety. I will discuss this in more detail below.

Second, case studies help locate the point being made in the real world. Quoting scientific studies showing something works may often feel very abstract or theory-based. Adding a case study helps remind us that an idea is real and relevant to our lives.

Making it relevant makes it easier to remember. I still recall a speech by Carrie Poppy as QED 2013 titled "In Defence of Anecdotes"[4]. In it, she wanted to make the point that ghosts do not exist and if you feel the presence of one, there is most likely a better explanation.

She could have done a try and boring talk about how the laws of physics do not allow for ghosts, shown the statistics on how common minor hallucinations are and brought in some studies supporting the idea that people imagine them. We all knew all of this of course.

Instead, she told us a story about the time she thought her apartment was haunted. Every time she spent time at home she began to feel cold and ill. There was a feeling she could not put her finger on, and gradually even her scepticism began to fade, and she wondered if there really was a ghost.

Then, one day, she posted about her experience online, and someone replied "have you checked for carbon monoxide poisoning?" Sure enough, when she did, she found her boiler had been slowly poisoning her by releasing carbon monoxide. I still remember this story long after I have forgotten all of the graphs and charts I saw that weekend. Case studies help us remember.

Why is reinforcement necessary?

In a perfect world, someone could tell us something once, and we would learn it and never forget it. We would take it on board immediately and start using that piece of knowledge.

---

4 Carrie Poppy. In Defence of Anecdotes. QED 2013.
https://www.youtube.com/watch?v=g9677GQocFw

However, anyone living in the real world knows this is not how humans work. Even when the stakes are high, we often fail to do this. People say "learn from your mistakes" you fail to take into account just how difficult this is. We fall into the same traps time and time again.

This problem is especially true of anxiety. If you have been reinforcing the same anxious thought patterns for years, or decades, they are not going to go away overnight.

There is a therapy technique used in anxiety called *exposure*. This is where you expose yourself to your phobia to see that it is safe and your anxiety is irrational. Of course, we already *know* our worry is irrational. It is making ourselves believe it that is the tricky bit.

This is the reason why exposure breaks the task down into several steps and repeats each step over and over again. If you had a phobia of chairs, you might start by just touching a chair. You would do this every day for weeks until you felt more comfortable, before moving on to sitting in the chair. The message that it is safe and you do not need to worry needs to be reinforced over and over again.

Intellectually, you know that it is irrational but getting your body to believe it takes time and reinforcement. Therefore, if you find I do repeat myself and say the same thing with case studies, remind yourself that this is not a mistake and this is not a waste of time. Intellectually, you know that this is just reinforcement, but it will nevertheless help your body take the message on board.

It is not often easy

I use the term *muggles* to refer to non-anxious folk. I think this analogy is apt because they are just like us, except that we have this hidden world within their world that is filled with anxiety.

One of the struggles with anxiety is that it makes doing everyday things more difficult. This means that making positive changes can be doubly difficult. Sleeping well and exercising more is something muggles struggle with, let alone when you are doing it with anxiety. So do not be too hard on yourself if you do not hit your goals first time. This stuff is difficult for everyone.

However, the rewards are worth it. Almost anything that is worth doing is hard. Otherwise, it would just be *the way*. Success comes to those who are willing to put in the work. To those who are willing to dedicate the time and effort needed to improve their lives. Step-by-step, we can make improvements.

Ready to go?

There are changes that you can make to your lifestyle to reduce your anxiety and improve your quality of life. This book will help you make them. Let's begin the journey.

Why focus on lifestyle?

This book looks at the changes you can make to your lifestyle to make yourself feel better. Before we get into the details of that, it is worth asking why we would want to.

For instance, why do we not just focus on curing our anxiety instead? Or why not focus on using specific therapy techniques, such as mindfulness, to help control our anxiety?

Some of these are great options. You may want to pursue them, and indeed some of my other books may help you do this. However, this book I want to focus solely on lifestyle. In this chapter, I will explain why and build the case for its importance.

There is no "cure" for anxiety

As I will explain in more detail in a later chapter, everyone has anxiety. It is a normal human emotion. In fact, it is crucial. Without it, we would stand in the middle of tracks, watching the oncoming train, without a care in the world.

Therefore, when we talk about managing or controlling anxiety, what we mean is that we want to bring it down to a healthy, manageable level. We want to stop it from preventing us doing the things we want to do with our life.

This is different from say a chest infection. Here we have a bacterial infection, and we take some antibiotics to get rid of it. Afterwards, it is gone we are back to just being us. With anxiety, this *is* us. There is nothing to remove: we just need to re-programme the software.

If we accept this principle, the issue then becomes how we can reduce our anxiety down to this level. There are a number of options to do this, and one is by using therapy and "cures". However, using an anxiety-friendly lifestyle can also be an effective way of doing this. The evidence suggests it is just as useful.

It is a good prescription

Everyone is banging on the drum of leading healthier, more active lifestyles. This is not an alternative to seeking treatment: it can be treatment itself. It is not unknown for doctors to prescribe going outside and exercising to patients with anxiety and depression.

That is because it has clinically proven benefits5. Healthy lifestyles benefit both the mind and the body.

It can run alongside treatment

Some treatments for anxiety are incompatible. Therapists might not accept you as a patient for cognitive behavioural therapy if you were already pursuing psychotherapy, for example. They would not want their work to interfere with each other.

There is no such concern for making changes to your lifestyle. Nobody is going to complain that you have started to build a stronger support network or eat healthier. In fact, they will probably be encouraging you to do so.

It is medication free

I am not one that likes to engage in the naturalistic fallacy. That is the idea that everything natural is good. I like science, evidence-based medicine and making full use of the last few thousand years of progress in a civilised society.

However, it is no secret that anti-anxiety medication such as selective serotonin reuptake inhibitors (SSRIs) can come with some significant side-effects. These side-effects are common: one study concluded that 38% of patients experienced side-effects, of which a quarter were classified as "very bothersome" or "extremely bothersome"6.

In comparison, there is no mediation required when making lifestyle changes. I would say that it is side-effect free, but if you are going to start pumping your guns at the gym every day, there might be some aching. For maximum gain, there is usually some pain.

5 Knapen J & Vancampfort D (2013). Evidence for exercise therapy in the treatment of depression and anxiety. International Journal of Psychosocial Rehabilitation. Vol 17(2) 75-87

6 Elisa Cascade, Amir H. Kalali, MD, and Sidney H. Kennedy, MD, FRCPC. Real-World Data on SSRI Antidepressant Side Effects. Psychiatry (Edgmont). 2009 Feb; 6(2): 16–18.

It is accessible, and often free

Therapy can often be difficult to obtain. Even if your country as a universal healthcare system, the chances are that there will be a waiting list for such options. You also have the option to seek private help, which can be accessed much faster, but typically at a high price.

In the UK, estimates for private therapy vary. The British Association for Counselling and Psychotherapy place the amount at £10-£50 per session, while the NHS suggests psychotherapy will cost between £40-£100 per hour.

Let's say we take a middle estimate of £50 per hour. Therapy can often take a year to be effective7. 52 weekly sessions at £50 each comes to £2,600. This amount of money is simply out-of-reach to many people.

In comparison, there are no waiting lists, and often no costs associated with making changes to your lifestyle.

You do not need to speak to your GP or get anyone's permission to make changes. You can just make them, or at least try to. You can get started as soon as you are ready to.

Often, these changes will come at no cost. Sometimes there will be, or at least the option to involve spending money, but some changes can be made without any additional spending. Some even reduce the amount of money you are spending already.

It comes with all-around benefits

Leading a healthier, more active lifestyle is good for your physical health as well as your mental health8. That might sound obvious because physical health benefits are what we associate with clean living.

---

7 S. SIMPSON, R. CORNEY, P. FITZGERALD and J. BEECHAM. A randomized controlled trial to evaluate the effectiveness and cost-effectiveness of psychodynamic counselling for general practice patients with chronic depression. Psychological Medicine, Volume 33, Issue 2. February 2003, pp. 229-239. DOI: http://dx.doi.org/10.1017/S0033291702006517

8 Darren E.R. Warburton, Crystal Whitney Nicol, and Shannon S.D. Bredin. Health benefits of physical activity: the evidence. CMAJ. 2006 Mar 14; 174(6): 801-809. doi: 10.1503/cmaj.051351

However, I think it is worth considering what the implications are for anxiety:

- You will feel better9. Leading a healthier lifestyle is a strong predictor of how happy you will be.
- It helps stabilise your mood10. If you experience ups and downs, which almost everyone with anxiety does, you may find these highs and lows are less pronounced after making changes to your lifestyle.
- You will be ill less often11. This means less minor illness, less feeling rubbish, less sulking around at home while you wait for a cold to clear up.
- You reduce the chance of serious illness12. Serious illness often leads to more anxiety and depression13, so anything we can do to mitigate the risk is a positive step.

These examples come from specific changes you can make to your lifestyle, and I will go into more detail about each of these in later chapters. This list provides a nice summary of the benefits, and I am sure you will agree that these are worth having.

It provides life-long benefits

Therapy may provide significant short-term benefits, but it could also be that the long-term benefits are less significant14. Some people find they need to have some top-up periodically to maintain the benefit.

---

9 Germán Lobosa, Marcos Morab, María del Carmen Lapoc, Constanza Caligaria, Berta Schnettlerd. Happiness and health and food-related variables: Evidence for different age groups in Chile. Suma Psicológica. Volume 22, Issue 2, July–December 2015, Pages 120–128. DOI: http://dx.doi.org/10.1016/j.sumpsi.2015.09.002

10 Lane AM1, Lovejoy DJ. The effects of exercise on mood changes: the moderating effect of depressed mood. J Sports Med Phys Fitness. 2001 Dec;41(4):539-45.

11 NHS Choices. Preventing colds and flu. 13 October 2014. http://www.nhs.uk/Livewell/coldsandflu/Pages/Preventionandcure.aspx

12 World Health Organization. Diet, nutrition and the prevention of chronic diseases: Report of the joint WHO/FAO expert consultation. WHO Technical Report Series, No. 916 (TRS 916).

13 G. Rodin, MD, M. Katz, MD, N. Lloyd, BSc, E. Green, RN BScN MSc(T), J.A. Mackay, MA MSc, and R.K.S. Wong, MB ChB MSc, the Supportive Care Guidelines Group of Cancer Care Ontario's Program in Evidence-Based Care. Treatment of depression in cancer patients. Curr Oncol. 2007 Oct; 14(5): 180–188.

This in itself is reasonable. Many medical conditions require management and you may find you need to boost your treatment from time to time.

However, making lasting lifestyle changes can be an alternative to this. Once you incorporate positive changes into your lifestyle, they form part of who you are and are maintainable for the rest of your life.

Even temporary changes can have lasting benefits. For example, adult learning (completing a course as an adult) can have benefits that stay around for years or even decades after the course has finished15.

It is socially acceptable

I am very positive about how society views mental health. The evidence shows that attitudes continue to improve over both the short and long term16.

70% of people now feel confident talking to their friends and family about their mental health issues17. Of course, that means 30%, one in three, do not. If you are in that 30%, that is centirely understandable.

It can be awkward, uncomfortable or embarrassing to say to people "I am starting antidepressants next week" or "I will be in late on Wednesday because I have cognitive behavioural therapy". You may feel like you have to hide what you are doing, or simply do not feel discussing it with the people who would typically provide you with emotional support.

Making changes to your lifestyle does not have this problem. Living healthier comes with none of the stigmas and is actively encouraged by the rest of the society. Your friends and family will probably be excited to hear about the changes that you have made and provide you with valuable support and encouragement.

---

14 Paykel ES, Scott J, Cornwall PL, et al. Duration of relapse prevention after cognitive therapy in residual depression: follow-up of controlled trial. Psychological Med 2005;35:59–68.

15 Mental Health Today, "The impact of adult and community learning programmes on mental health and wellbeing", https://is.gd/XOkkII

16 Time to Change. Attitudes to Mental Illness 2014 Research Report. April 2015.

17 NHS Information Centre. Attitudes to Mental Illness - 2011 survey report. 8 June 2011.

As it is something that muggles do, non-anxious friends and family may also be able to offer advice and information based on their experiences doing similar things.

Case study

Paul was too embarrassed to talk to his friends about his anxiety. He would spend all the time worrying and felt awkward in social situations. However, he also worried that his friends would not be supportive if he was honest about this.

Instead, he decided to use lifestyle to improve his anxiety. He set up a regular fitness routine where he would meet a friend at the gym and they would work out together.

It was hard work, but Paul benefited from having a friend there without having to discuss his anxiety with anyone.

There is a lot of options and support

Not only is it something that is socially acceptable to the people you know, but wider society as a whole has a tonne of support for such changes, too.

Everyone is on the bandwagon of healthier living. Most healthcare providers have a range of support options and advice, and society is overrun with groups and businesses looking to support people's efforts.

Want to exercise more? There are gyms, running clubs and sports teams. Want to eat healthier? There are recipes online, NHS booklets and TV shows about cooking. Want to connect more and build a wider circle of friends? There are thousands of social groups in most cities.

It is fun

One of the best things about using lifestyle to manage your anxiety is that the process can be enjoyable.

Using therapy to tackle your anxiety is hard work and emotionally draining. Often, when you start a series of therapy sessions, your mood will go down before it comes up. This is because you are giving more focus to your anxiety and engaging with it. This reduction in mood is worth it if it gets results, but does make the process difficult.

In contrast, making positive changes to your lifestyle can be an enjoyable and exciting process. You get to do new things, things which may not be anxiety-provoking in themselves, and still make yourself feel better.

Summary

Developing an anxiety-friendly lifestyle is an excellent way to manage and reduce your anxiety. It can be used alongside therapy and treatment, has few side-effects, is clinically proven to work and can be fun and exciting to do.

Understanding anxiety

Before I talk about how you can change your lifestyle to improve your anxiety, we need a basic grounding on what anxiety is and how it relates to us. Doing this will give us a framework for understanding what we are doing and why we are doing it.

Anxiety is a normal human emotion

It may sometimes feel like you have all the anxiety and everyone around you has none. This is not the case. Everyone has some degree of anxiety because it is a normal human emotion that we all feel.

Anxiety is part of our evolution. It is a survival technique. It keeps us safe from harm. Without it we would walk into dangerous situations and not bother to get ourselves out of them. Therefore, when we talk about "fixing" anxiety, we do not want to get rid of it, we merely want to bring it down to a manageable level.

Fight or flight

Anxiety comes from the fight or flight response. This is a deep-down response from the brain whenever it senses danger: do we fight off the threat or do we run away?

Humans evolved in a time before most threats were hidden behind cages and yellow safety tape. When primitive humans (or any animal) sees a threat it has to respond. When we see a lion in the grass in front of us, for example, our body gets ready to fight or flee.

What happens from a physiological perspective? Our body starts diverting blood flow and energy away from systems less essential to fighting or fleeing, such as the brain or digestive system, and towards muscles.

This response is the reason we can experience an increased heart rate and symptoms such as stomach discomfort, light-headedness and rapid breathing.

False positives and negatives

Anxiety is a survival mechanism set up to keep us safe. The human body is wired to be over cautious because that is the best strategy for keeping us alive.

Consider the following scenario: there may or may not be a deadly snake slivering through the grass. There are four ways this could play out.

	There is a snake	There is no snake
We run away	Positive identification. We run away and successfully escape a deadly snake attack.	False positive. We run away for no reason.
We do not run away	False negative. We get killed by a deadly snake.	Nothing happens.

In the first row, we get scared and run away. This is very useful if there is a snake. We can avoid a potentially deadly attack. If there is no snake, not much harm is done either. We have run away for no reason, which leaves us feeling out of breath and maybe a bit silly, but otherwise unharmed.

In the second row, we do not run away. This action is fine if there is no snake, but if there is one, we are risking an attack. Not running away has very severe consequences.

Therefore, when Mother Nature came to evolve us into the ultimate survival machines, she decided to play it safe. It was much better for us to have a fear system that triggered easily and played it safe, than one that did not.

Our brain is designed to panic first and think later because the consequences of panicking are minor from a survival point of view (though highly uncomfortable in the modern world) and the consequences of not panicking are severe.

How the brain works

We tend to think of the brain as one single unit. After all, we tend to think of our brain as "us". We are our brain. We see it as one unit that does all of our thinking, and controls our actions.

This is just the case. Our brain is lots of different systems grouped together. Most of the time the systems work as one, and we enjoy a coherent experience of the world. However, all too often, they come into conflict with each other.

Think of your body like a city. A city is full of citizens, just like your body has lots of parts. A city is nominally run by the local government, just like your body is run by the brain.

Here are some observations about how a government runs a city:

- The city was not designed to some grand plan (unless you live in Milton Keynes18) but evolved over time with new developments built on top of old developments.
- The old developments were not necessarily removed, and may still be used to greater or lesser extents.
- The government sets the rules, and most of the time the citizens follow them.
- Sometimes the citizens do not follow the rules, and there is not much the government can do about it.
- The government has multiple departments, who do not always talk to each other and sometimes come into conflict.
- The government is often reacting to what the citizens are doing, rather than proactively setting the agenda.
- The whole thing is a bit of a mess.

Our body is the same. Our brain is usually in control of what is going on. This is not always the case, though. Sometimes a part of the body decides to do something different, and all the brain can do is react to what is going on. Sometimes different parts of the brain have different opinions and have to fight it out with each other.

In The Happiness Hypothesis19, author Jonathan Haidt uses the analogy of the elephant and the rider. Our higher brain functions are the rider. Most of the time, the rider can steer the elephant in the diction they want to go. However, when the elephant gets spooked and decides to run, there is not much the rider can do.

Systems in conflict

When it comes to anxiety, there are two key systems in the brain that are relevant. One is the prefrontal cortex. This is where our higher reasoning lives. It is responsible for planning, impulse control and rational thinking.

---

18 The Plan for Milton Keynes. Milton Keynes Development Corporation. March 1970. ISBN 0-903379-00-7.

19 Jonathan Haidt. The Happiness Hypothesis: Finding Modern Truth in Ancient Wisdom. 26 December 2006. ISBN: 0465028020.

The other is the amygdala. This is part of the limbic system and plays a significant part in triggering our fear response[20]. It does not have the higher reasoning your prefrontal cortex has but does have control over the fight or flight response lever.

This is why anxiety can feel pretty silly. Your prefrontal cortex is well aware that there is no danger from that apple in front of you and that your apple phobia is completely irrational. Your amygdala is not interested, though. It senses danger and has no plans to take its hand off the panic lever.

Anxiety feedback cycle

One of the reasons it can be so difficult to conquer anxiety is because feeling anxious promotes the idea that there is something wrong, which in itself breeds more anxiety.

When we experience symptoms of anxiety, these combine with negative thoughts. This can cause us to focus more on how we feel. We then notice the symptoms of anxiety even more, interpret this with a negative bias and therefore make the symptoms even worse.

This process is called the anxiety feedback cycle.

20 Justin S. Feinstein, Ralph Adolphs, Antonio Damasio, Daniel Tranell. The Human Amygdala and the Induction and Experience of Fear. Current Biology. Volume 21, Issue 1, 11 January 2011, Pages 34–38. DOI: http://dx.doi.org/10.1016/j.cub.2010.11.042

ANXIETY FEEDBACK CYCLE

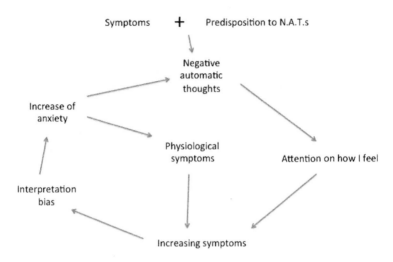

A powerful defence against anxiety is to recognise that we are in this feedback cycle. When you do not know why you are feeling this way, it is easy to add a negative interpretation to the feeling. However, if you can identify it is anxiety, it helps us understand why we are feeling this way, and thus help us break out of the feedback cycle.

Case study

Susan suffered from health anxiety. Whenever she felt unwell, she convinced herself it was cancer. This thought would make her feel even worse, reinforcing the physical symptoms she was already feeling and sent her into a downward spiral.

After reading a book on anxiety that explained about the feedback cycle, she decided to draw a copy out. Then, each time she began feeling ill, she would look at the diagram she had drawn.

She still worried she had cancer. However, because she could see the way in which anxiety made her feel worse, she felt reassured that some of the bad feeling was anxiety, rather than serious illness. This thought made her feel a little better.

Expectations vs reality

Anxiety is a memory disorder. Your memory will trick you, and it will lie to you. It does not matter how many times you have been in a crowded room and not exploded; your memory will not supply that evidence during a panic attack.

This is also true of doing tasks that will make you feel better. Your memory will not surface those memories of how good it felt to see your friend or go for a run. All you will feel is the negatives.

Let's take the example of going for a run. You think that you do not want to go for a run because it will be unpleasant. You feel fine now but when you start running it will be tiring, and you will ache, and your mood will be low. You think "I do not want to feel worse than I do now".

The reality is that the opposite will happen. Your mood is lowest before you go for the run. When you start running, and when you come back, your mood improves. We know this is the case and later on, we will look at the evidence showing us this is the case.

However, even though we know this is the case academically, our anxious mind steps in and says "no, you will feel worse, stay here and wallow".

This graph shows how we think we will feel when we are sitting around at home before a run:

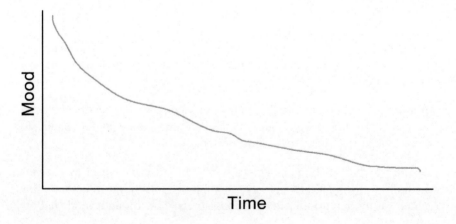

In reality this is how we feel when we go for a run:

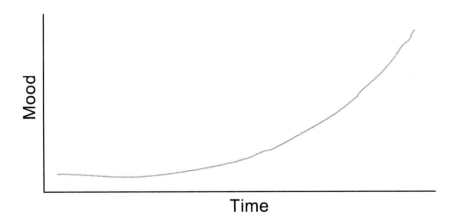

Time

This pattern is not just true for exercise. It is true **for everything**. When we think about going to see a friend or family member, we go through the same process. We tell ourselves it will be too much effort and yet when we do see them, we experience a mood uplift.

Regardless of the scenario, it is the same process. Our memory tells us that it will be unrewarding and to stay where we are when in fact just the opposite is true.

I will refer to this as *the memory trap*, and we will come back to it later on.

My memory traps

I usually go for a run on a Saturday morning. Sometimes, when I wake up, I feel uneasy on my stomach. I start to think "maybe I should skip today". This is the time I have to remind myself that going will make me feel better: and it does! Every time without fail.

It is not just exercise. When I think about going to my public speaking club or cooking a labour-intensive meal, I sometimes find myself weighing up the pros and cons, even though I know I always enjoy it when I get into it.

CBT and exposure

Cognitive behavioural therapy (CBT) has emerged as one of the leading methods to treat anxiety. It looks at both your thinking (the cognitive side) and your actions (the behavioural side).

CBT identifies errors in your thoughts and then puts them to the test. For example, let's say you struggled with social anxiety and hated going to parties before you were worried you would be embarrassed.

The way CBT would approach this is to say "what are the chances of this happening?" and "what are the social costs if it did happen?". Asking these questions allows us to identify the following errors in our thinking:

- We think the probability of it happening is high, but in reality, it is unlikely that we will embarrass ourselves.
- We think it will be the end of the world if we embarrass ourselves, but in reality, nobody will notice. Or, if they do, we can just laugh it off. It will be upsetting, but not fatal.

We then go out and test these predictions with experiments. These exercises are where exposure kicks in.

Exposure

Exposure is the process of putting yourself in uncomfortable situations to demonstrate to your anxiety that they are not as bad as you think they are. For example, if you struggle with social anxiety, going to a party would be a classic example.

Sounds scary, right?

Do not fear: we use a technique called ***graded*** exposure. This is the process of breaking a process down into smaller, manageable chunks. You create a hierarchy of tasks and work through them, starting with the easiest and building up. There is no rush to progress: you can repeat one level as many times as you like.

Let's take the social anxiety about parties example again. What would a graded exposure hierarchy look like for this?

Fear (1-100)	Activity
100	Going to a party by myself and staying all night.
90	Going to a party by myself and staying for 1 hour.
80	Going to a party by myself and staying for 30 minutes.
70	Going to a party with friends and staying all night.
60	Going to a party with friends and staying for 1 hour.
50	Going to a party with one friend and staying all night.
40	Going to a party with one friend and staying for 1 hour.

30	Going to a party where I know everybody.
20	Going to see a few friends.
10	Going to see one friend and staying for 1 hour.

We start with a very manageable task: hanging out with a friend for one hour. We then slowly build up to harder tasks. At each level, we feel slightly uncomfortable, but it does not feel out of our reach. If it does, we break the task down into smaller chunks.

Over time, this allows us to achieve things that we thought would be impossible.

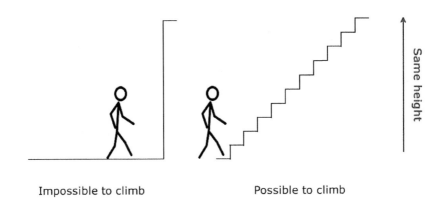

Impossible to climb   Possible to climb

I discuss exposure in much more detail in my book **Technical Anxiety**[21]. For this book, we have now covered enough to get going.

Case study

Samantha hated eating in restaurants. She was worried everyone was watching her while she ate. Soon, she stopped going out for dinner at all. Doing this meant missing out on social events and birthday celebrations with friends.

She started an online CBT programme that helped her develop a fear hierarchy to use for exposure therapy. She broke the tasks down step-by-

---

21 Chris Worfolk. Technical Anxiety: The complete guide to what is anxiety and what to do about it. ISBN: 978-1539424215

step, starting with an easy-to-escape fast food restaurant and then moving on to formal sit-down meals.

1. Go to a fast food restaurant and get a drink to take away
2. Go to a fast food restaurant and get a meal to take away
3. Go to a fast food restaurant and get a drink to eat in
4. Go to a fast food restaurant and get a meal to drink in
5. Go to a fast food restaurant and eat in with a friend
6. Go to a quiet hotel restaurant and eat lunch by yourself
7. Go to a quiet hotel restaurant and eat lunch with a friend
8. Go to a busy restaurant and eat dinner

She had to repeat some of the steps several times before she felt comfortable enough to move on to the next step. However, eventually, she worked her way through the entire list and was able to join her friends.

Why is this important?

I will make references to CBT and exposure throughout the rest of the book. It is a useful technique when we find ourselves with a task we do not think we can complete. Therefore, it is important that we both understand what t means when I talk about exposure.

Summary

In this chapter, we reminded ourselves that anxiety is a normal human emotion that everyone experiences. We looked at how fight or flight works and learnt that the brain is a set of different systems that do not always work together as well as we would hope.

We discovered that our memory lies to us and that it is important to remember this when we are struggling for motivation. Finally, we learnt about graded exposure, and how breaking a task down makes it easier to complete.

You can change

One of the biggest struggles against anxiety is fighting against our mind's natural resistance to change. It is easy to give up, or simply never start something, because we feel that it will inevitably end in failure.

In this chapter, I want to build the case that this is not true and explain how to overcome such feelings. We will look at why people often fail to reach their objectives, anxiety or no anxiety, and what they are doing wrong.

Our flexible brains

I often speak about the problem that evolution has left us. Our brains evolved over hundreds of thousands of years. They are designed to keep us alive long enough to reproduce at a time when we were hunter-gatherers. Now we put our brains in offices, planes and night clubs and wonder why they are confused.

Such thoughts often paint a gloomy picture. If our brains were never designed to cope with modern life, perhaps they will never be able to adapt (in our lifetime).

I am more positive about the situation. Our brains have been doing an excellent job. We think of change as a relatively recent thing because the pace of change is ever increasing. However, change has been around a long time.

Compared to our hunter gatherer days, society has been rapidly changing since we discovered agriculture 5,000 years ago. Since then we have transitioned from our traditional way of life to one that is unrecognisable to any other species on Earth. Yet we have done it and done it with ease.

Many people feel anxious about travelling, cities, being at home, work, relationships and many other things. But few of us feel anxious about all of them. In the case of general anxiety disorder (GAD), most of us are worried about the unknowns of the future, not the strange world of the present.

The reason we can cope, which we all are to some extent, is that Mother Nature gave us a brain that could adapt. Here is how neuroscientist Jack Gallant, head of the Gallant Lab at UC Berkeley, puts it22.

---

22 Jack Gallent. This Is Your Brain on Podcasts. Freakonomics Podcast. 12 October 2016.

"We kind of have a fixed brain, but during development, and even when we're adults, we can learn to flexibly use that system to solve novel problems. That doesn't say the system can't be overwhelmed or confused or operate sub-optimally, but it's a pretty damn flexible system."

Our brains can comphrend the modern scary world. It is harder for some people than others, and harder at certain times rather than others, but it is an amazingly adaptable system.

Epigenetics

Our DNA plays a large part in who we are. Steven Pinker suggests that around 50% of our personality is genetic[23], and the other 50% is environmental[24].

If so much of our personality is controlled by our genes, does that mean we are stuck with it? It certainly could seem like a genetic predisposition to anxiety could make it more difficult for some of us.

That is the key word, though. It is *more* difficult: not impossible. Our genetics only accounts for half of our personality and the other half we can shape with our environment.

This is where the field of *epigenetics* comes in. We can think of our genes as the hardware of our bodies. Our genes do not change: we are stuck with those for life. However, that is only half the story. The other half is the software that is running on top of this hardware. This we can change, and epigenetics is studying how and why this happens.

The causation myth

On the face of it, anxiety seems simple. You are in a situation that makes you feel uncomfortable, which causes you to have anxious thoughts. These cause unpleasant feelings, which then leads to symptoms of anxiety.

This view is how we see the world in general. We have thoughts, and those thoughts trigger feelings and actions. We are autonomous beings with free will.

---

23 Steven Pinker. How the Mind Works. 17 January 1999. ISBN: 0393318486

24 Steven Pinker. How the Mind Works. 17 January 1999. ISBN: 0393318486

This concept was the premise behind cognitive therapy. The idea was that if we could intervene at the cognitive level, we could stop people from having the anxious feelings, and therefore their problems would be solved.

The problem is that cognitive therapy did not work. It was only when a behavioural aspect was added, to form cognitive behavioural therapy, that we started to see results.

Why is it that intervening at the behavioural level succeeded when intervening at the cognitive level did not? Could it be that there is something wrong with our model of causation?

Reversing the arrow

While most of the world was happy with the idea of feelings following thoughts, the nineteenth-century academic and psychology pioneer William James was not. He argued that we had it the wrong way round.

Instead of us smiling because we were feeling happy, James argued that we felt happy because we smiled.

The idea that our feelings follow our actions, and not our thoughts, was summed up in a 2012 book by psychologist Richard Wiseman, entitled **Rip It Up**25. The book summarises many scenarios in which our feelings seem to follow our actions, rather than our thoughts.

Case study

David suffered from depression. He had been referred for CBT but, unfortunately, his therapist was entirely focused on the cognitive aspects. They looked at how to challenge unwanted thoughts.

The problem was that David did not have unwanted thoughts: he would simply wake up feeling like he could not face the world. The thoughts came later, but they were not there to greet him when he first opened his eyes.

In his second round of CBT, his new therapist was far more focused on the behavioural side of CBT. His therapist encouraged him to set up a morning routine, where he would get up at a set time, have breakfast and walk the dog.

---

25 Richard Wiseman. Rip It Up: Forget positive thinking, it's time for positive action. 5 July 2012. ISBN: 1447273362

Now, when David woke up with the feelings, he did not have to challenge them. He would simply follow his routine if he could. He found that when he forced himself, he felt much better afterwards. Some days he could not force himself to, and that was okay too: he was making improvements slowly.

What is the impact for anxiety?

The idea that feelings may come from actions is great news for designing an anxiety-friendly lifestyle.

I have already put forward the case that developing such a lifestyle it worthwhile in itself. You will improve your physical health, it is a fun thing to do and has clinically proven benefits for your mental health. These benefits alone would make it worth doing.

However, the idea of actions driving our anxiety adds another layer.

When you go through a rough patch and find yourself rarely exercising, eating poorly and not looking after yourself, you may see it as a consequence of anxiety.

That is exactly how it feels at the time. If I am feeling low my adherence to a proper diet and regular exercise fades fast. The motivation to follow a proper sleep schedule and interact with other people is sapped from me.

This is exactly how it feels at the time. However, if we accept the causation arrow goes the other way, that means that our feelings can be driven by our actions, and therefore if we force ourselves to do the correct actions, we can make ourselves feel better and reduce our anxiety.

Good behaviours will lead our anxious thoughts and feelings to reduce.

Too good to be true?

To some, this may sound too good to be true. The idea that all we need to do is change our actions and we will magically stop feeling anxious is a big claim to make.

In fact, it sounds downright silly. You might as well say "oh just do the thing you are afraid of and you will feel better about it afterwards". This may or may not be the case, but if we could just do everything we wanted to do, we would not be sat here wondering how to control our anxiety.

Luckily, we can avoid this issue because this is not the claim I am making. However, this situation is subtly different from confronting your anxiety head on. We are not putting ourselves in high anxiety situations. We are making positive lifestyle changes that are fun to implement.

Second, I am not claiming this will "cure" your anxiety. As we have discussed there is nothing to **cure**, it is that we want to reduce it to a manageable level.

Third, there is nothing "quick-fix" about this idea. Making lasting and meaningful changes takes a long time. Making positive changes will often make us feel good straight away. However, to see a reduction in anxiety we will have to work on a much wider timescale.

Case study

Tina had struggled with her weight since early adulthood. She experienced a lot of social anxiety at work. She knew she should eat healthier, but by the time she got home at night, she would often feel so drained that she would abandon her plans for a healthy meal and order a pizza instead.

When she overheard someone calling her "fat", she decided it was time to do something about it. She joined a local diet group for support and began to change her eating habits.

Progress was slow at first: it was easy to fall back to eating junk food. Tina started counting the number of healthy meals she had and set herself a target of increasing the number each month. She recorded the results in a diary.

Slowly, she found that the number of healthy meals increased. She also found that she had more energy during the day and found it easier to face the world. As her mood increased, she felt more motivated to cook on an evening, and therefore found it easier to continue with her new eating habits.

A history of change

Remember that anxiety is a memory disorder (you did **remember** that, right?). Your memory lies to you. When you think about changing, you may experience the negative automatic thought (NAT) "I cannot change".

Is this real, or is this your memory lying to you?

Technically, it could be either. However, I have yet to meet **anyone** who falls into column one. The idea that you cannot change is merely a NAT.

In fact, my guess is that if you look back at your life, without the cloud anxiety, you will see that you have changed. Where you the same one year? Ten years ago? Probably not, right? You have changed, grown, learnt.

Maybe you feel less anxious than you used to. Maybe you feel **more** anxious than you used to. Maybe your anxiety has changed. Even if you feel you are more anxious than you used to be, that is still a change. And if you can change one way, you can change the other way.

Reflection exercise

Take a moment now to consider how you have changed over the past 1-10 years. What is different? How is your anxiety different? Better yet, write it down.

Ask yourself the following questions:

- How has the intensity of my anxiety changed over the past decade? Is it better or worse?
- How has the frequency changed over that time? Do I have more frequent or fewer panic attacks now? How about spells of intense worry?
- How have the subjects I am anxious about changed over that time? What did I used to worry about that I do not worry about now? What new worries have I picked up?
- How has me behaviour changed over that time? Are there things I do now that I did not do back then?
- How have my coping mechanisms changed over that time? What do I do about my anxiety now? How do I feel about it?

The last question is particularly important. There are things you do to reduce or face up to your anxiety that I am guessing you did not do ten years ago. Recently, you bought this book, for example. Why did you buy it now, and not a year ago? How has your relationship with anxiety changed?

Recording exercise

Here is another useful exercise to do. Answer the same questions but in the present tense.

- How intense is my anxiety?
- How frequently do I have panic attacks or intense worry?
- What am I worrying about?
- What do I do about it? What do I avoid?

- What are my coping mechanisms?
- What am I doing to tackle my anxiety?
- How do I feel about my anxiety?

Write it down on paper, then put it in an envelope for safekeeping. Review it in a year's time, then again in five years and ten years. If you do not believe what I am saying about change now, you will when you review the letter.

But it does not feel like I have changed!

I have repeatedly stressed the idea that change happens slowly. You do not go to a motivational seminar and change your life: if that were possible, you would get them on prescription from your doctor. Instead, change happens gradually over time.

What do we know about gradual changes? We do not notice them.

I think about the sun. It travels across the sky every day. When you wake up it is on one side; when you go to bed it is on the other. But, even if you sat and watched the sun, it would never appear to move26.

Similarly, we do not notice changes in ourselves or those that we see every day. If you have been around babies, you will know that they change so fast. Week to week they can look like different people. However, if you are a parent, you will also notice that they never seem to change.

When my daughter was born, my parents would come round to see her every Saturday. And every Saturday they would say the same thing: "I can't believe how much she has changed since last week." But, because I saw her every day, I could never see the change. For me, it was gradual, for them it was discrete. It is only when I look back at photos that I can see the difference.

Guess what? You are living your life 24/7, so you never notice the changes either. They are gradual. It is only by looking back that you will be able to see how much you have changed.

---

26 Unless you live on the equator, in which case, you can see it moving around sunrise and sunset.

The compound effect

At this stage, you might be thinking "okay, maybe people can make small changes - but not big ones". You know what? Even if that is the case, it does not matter. We can use something called *the compound effect* to get the results we want.

In these terms, compound is originally a financial word. It is the idea that when you earn interest, this is interest is put back into your bank account. The next year, not only are you earning interest on your original investment, but you are also earning interest on the interest you have already earned. This feature is called *compound interest*.

How much is it worth? Let's say you put £1,000 in a savings account in 1980 and earned, on average, 5% interest per year. Without compound interest, that would be worth £2,850 today. With compound interest, it would be worth £6,081.

Scenario	Start	End	Gain
Without compound interest	£1,000	£2,850	£1,850
With compound interest	£1,000	£6,081	£5,081

You have gained nearly three times as much money with compound interest as without it. And it only goes up from there. The rate of growth continues to accelerate.

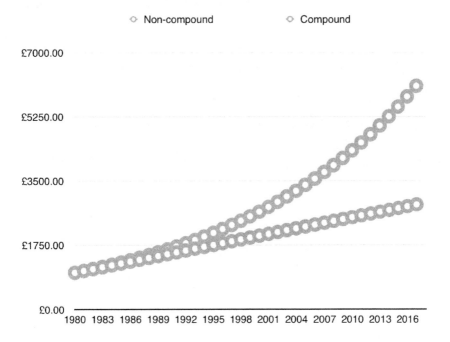

At first, the lines look the same. There is almost no difference. There are no massive changes here.

Lessons from compounding

They key point in compounding is that it does not require huge changes. Just be reinvesting the interest, we get small changes. At the end of year two, the difference is only £2.50. At the end of year three, the difference is only £7.63.

Over the long term, these little changes add up. By the end, it adds up to thousands of pounds, many times what we started with, and continues to grow exponentially.

Making changes in **your life** is the same. We do not need to make huge changes. We just need to persistently make small changes and wait for them to add up.

Summary

In this chapter, we learnt that we are born with a particular set of genes, but that does not mean we cannot change. By reprogramming our software using a behaviour-led series of small changes, we can reduce our anxiety and feel better.

However, it is easy to dismiss this evidence when you feel down. There is a difference between believing something academically and believing it wholeheartedly. To be honest, I do not *expect* a few sections on the science of behavioural change will instantly win you over.

But that is okay. Believing you can make big changes in your life is not essential at this stage. All I need is for you to be open to the idea that it *might* be possible. Then, when we start making changes, you will see it in action.

Techniques for change

In the previous chapter, we learnt that we ***could*** change. I know what you are you thinking: "all of that evidence sounds fine, but I have tried to change before, and I did not achieve the changes I wanted".

It's true; it is challenging, and sometimes we all fail. However, this time there will be a difference. We are going to go into battle armed with new techniques and new tools to help us change. In this chapter, we will learn these techniques, and in the next chapter, we will see how we can put them into a system that prevents us from failing.

Acknowledging the resistance

As we learnt in the chapter on understanding anxiety, one of the most robust defences have against worry is to acknowledge that we are trapped in the anxiety feedback cycle and recognise that it is anxiety that is making us feel this way.

The same thing can happen when trying to make a change in our life. As anxiety sufferers, we have a negative bias about situations. Therefore it is likely we tell ourselves we cannot change, even though there may be little evidence for it.

Once we get into this mindset, it makes us more likely to fail at the changes we want to make, which then combines with our negative bias to make it feel like change is impossible. I call this the change resistance cycle.

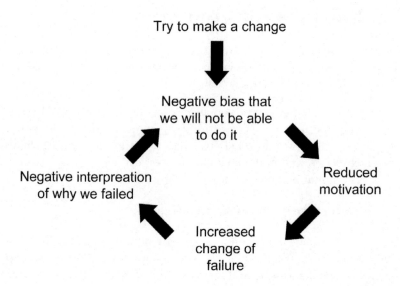

Try to make a change

Negative bias that
we will not be able
to do it

Reduced
motivation

Increased
change of
failure

Negative interpreation
of why we failed

There are two points we should take note of from this diagram.

The first is that having anxiety will make you feel like you cannot change. It is not that you actually cannot change, merely that your anxiety will make you feel this way. When you get the feeling that you cannot change, gently remind yourself that it is your anxiety talking.

The second is that even if you have failed to change in the past, this is still the anxiety talking. Because it saps your motivation when you do not recognise it for what it is, it has led to making it more difficult to change in the past. However, now we understand this, it will be easier to overcome this in the future.

Case study

Alex has always wanted to learn to speak basic Spanish. He signed up for an online course. It was tough: he struggled the remember the vocabulary and to pronounce the words correctly. Despite this, he was scoring good marks on the tests.

Every time he forgot a word he would tell himself "you are useless, you will never learn this". However, because he was aware of the resistance, he would remind himself "that is the kind of thought anxiety causes" and that it was not an accurate representation of the world.

This view did not make him feel much better, but he did give him enough strength to continue with the course.

Change resistance

It is not just anxiety sufferers that dislike change. Everyone seems to be wary of it. Whether it is sticking with the status-quo or doing the same thing because it has been around a long time, people prefer to go with what they know27.

Why do we fear change?

Like so many of our problems, our fear of change is probably a by-product of our evolution. Humanity did not develop in a world that changed much. The Earth was pretty much the same for thousands of years before we built towns and cities.

Our bodies are survival machines. They like things to be dependable and are subscribers to the adage "if it ain't broke, don't fix it".

In ***Thinking, Fast and Slow***28 author Daniel Kahneman notes that we fear losing something more than we value gaining it and that people have an endowment effect for what they already have, making it seem more valuable than items they do not have.

For example, in one study half of the participants were given a free coffee mug, and the other half were not. Each participant was asked how much they would buy or sell the mugs for. People consistently demanded a higher price to sell the mug than they were previously willing to pay to buy one.

Why is a mug suddenly more valuable once you own it? Because you fear losing it.

In the same way, we fear change because we do not want to lose what we already have. Even if we are unhappy with our life, we use the adage "better the Devil you know" to stick with what we have.

---

27 Scott Eidelman, Jennifer Pattershall, Christian S. Crandall. Longer is better. Journal of Experimental Social Psychology. Volume 46, Issue 6, November 2010, Pages 993–998. DOI: http://dx.doi.org/10.1016/j.jesp.2010.07.008

28 Daniel Kahneman. Thinking, Fast and Slow. 25 October 2011. ISBN: 0374275637

Change resistance is a major factor in most walks of life. The tech startup Amazon, now the largest retailer in the world29, has been successful often because they have taken risks and pioneered change. For example, launching ebooks even though it would cannibalise their print book business, or launching a diverse range of products including web hosting, tablets, streaming services, and a marketplace for buying and selling human labour30.

How did CEO Jeff Bezos persuade the company to embrace change so readily? He identified what he called the "institutional no"31 - the automatic reaction to reject ideas because we fear change. Bezos made everyone aware of it and replaced it with the "institutional yes"32.

That does not mean that we can just think positive and everything will be okay. It is no miracle cure. However, as Noreena Hertz explains in her book *Eyes Wide Open*33, identifying our unconscious biases is one of the most productive things we can do to tackle them.

We need to remind ourselves that we have a built-in bias against change and that this is our anxiety taking, not an accurate reflection of the situation.

Change is really hard

Sometimes people fail to make changes because they assume that changing should be easy. It almost never is.

People often start off with the best of intentions, then run into trouble, feel like they cannot do it, and then give up. This situation is understandable because change is tough. Often, it is far harder than we imagine before we begin.

---

29 Shannon Pettypiece. Amazon Passes Wal-Mart as Biggest Retailer by Market Value. Bloomberg. 23 July 2015.

30 Amazon Technical Turk, https://www.mturk.com/

31 Brad Stone. The Everything Store: Jeff Bezos and the Age of Amazon. 15 October 2013. ISBN: 0316219266

32 Julia Kirby and Thomas A. Stewart. The Institutional Yes. Harvard Business Review. October 2007 issue.

33 Noreena Hertz. Eyes Wide Open. 24 September 2013. ISBN: 0062268619

Much like acknowledging that we have a built-in resistance to change, we need to acknowledge that change is hard and we will want to give up. It is only by pushing through these feelings that we succeed.

Everything is more difficult when you have anxiety

Anxiety makes everything more difficult. For example, getting up and going for a run every morning is something that anyone would struggle with. Muggles find it hard, often impossible, to commit to.

Now, imagine doing all of that when you wake up filled with existential dread and a desire to hide under the covers. This is the challenge we have, right?

It is easy to slip into the mindset of "I cannot do this", but it is an even deeper hole to start thinking "I cannot do this even though everyone else can".

It is not that we are failures: it is that it is harder for us. The same amount of willpower does not go as far. Therefore, we need to be kind to ourselves and not chastise ourselves when something takes a little longer.

Summary of change resistance

Change is really tough. I am not selling you an easy system here: it requires hard work. It is important to remember that. As you try and make changes, you will run into setbacks, roadblocks and feelings that you cannot change.

When these arrive, you need to remind yourself:

- Change is tough and happens slowly
- Everyone struggles with change resistance, not just me
- Change is especially hard for me due to anxiety
- Anxiety causes my memory to lie to be amount what is possible
- I knew these feelings would come up, and I will push through them

Setting better goals

One of the reasons people in the wider world fail to hit targets is because the targets were badly designed. Spending time setting a good goal will make the difference between reaching it and failing to achieve it.

A lot of the advice in this chapter and the next boils down to setting better ones.

Setting SMART targets

In the business world, there is a concept known as **SMART targets**. SMART is an acronym with the following meaning:

Specific. It must be clear what you are going to do. Something vague like "exercise more" is hard to complete because when it comes to putting it into practice, there is no clear action. A much better goal would be "go for a run twice a week" because it is evident from the goal what you are going to do.

Measurable. How will you know if you have achieved it? For example "have a better diet" does not provide any metric by which you can measure how successful you are. Whereas "eat x number of vegetables each day" or "eat x number of calories" are much better because they are measurable: you can count how many you have eaten and therefore see how successful you have been and how that success rate changes over time.

Agreed. In business, this would refer to both the manager and the employee agreeing that the target as a good one and that they were both happy with it. In our personal lives, we are our own manager. Therefore, this step involves agreeing on a target with yourself.

Are you committed to achieving it? Do not select "go to the gym five times a week" if you have no intention of doing so, or are not excited enough to motivate yourself to carry it through. It is much better to put "go to the gym once a week" as a starting point, and then build it up once you have step one incorporated into your routine.

Realistic. The goal must be achievable. If you have been struggling with social anxiety disorder (SAD) for years, selecting a goal of "meeting a new person every day" is likely to be aiming a little high.

Remember that you can always exceed your goals, but failing to reach them hurts. You want to make the goal a challenge to push yourself, but make sure that it is a realistic goal that is not inevitably going to leave you feeling like a failure for not achieving it.

Time-based. Good goals have a specific period by which they need to be completed. Doing this provides a number of advantages. First, it provides you with some motivation. If you have a date you have to get it done by, it is less easy to tell yourself you can "just do it tomorrow".

Second, it prevents you from spending too much time on something that is not working. You might decide to do something every day for 60 days and see how it goes. At the end of the 60 days, if it works you can keep it, if not, it may be best to put the goal down as a learning exercise that did not work so well and move on to something else.

For the reasons outlined above, SMART targets are far better than fuzzy, unstructured targets. Whenever you set a goal, you should measure it against the SMART target criteria. If it does not measure up, alter it until it does.

Case study

Mark and Claire both wanted to increase their fitness.

Mark wrote a goal of "do more exercise". It was not a SMART goal. Every day he got up and told himself "I should do some exercise today" but would then think "oh, I can just do it tomorrow, when I have decided what I want to do". After a month, he still had not done anything.

Claire set a goal of "join a gym this week and go every Tuesday and Friday". Her plan was clear and measurable. At the end of the month, she had joined the gym and visited on all but one of the days she was supposed to.

Why did Claire succeed where Mark failed? Because the conversation she had with herself was different. Mark used up his mental energy working out the plan. Claire used her mental energy executing on the clear and actionable steps she had already laid down.

There must be clear actions

Setting a broad goal is an excellent way to work out where you want to get to in the long term. However, it is important to remember that you need to get up tomorrow and start doing it.

Let's say your goal is to climb Mount Everest. It is a big goal but an achievable one. The question is "how are you going to achieve it?" Where will you start? What will you do?

Each broad goal needs a set of actionable smaller goals that you can follow through on to lead you to your bigger goal. For example, if you did want to climb Mount Everest your milestone goals could be:

- Increase my climbing practice to twice per week
- Increase my cross training workouts to three times per week
- Complete a course on rope skills, rock falls, oxygen tanks, etc
- Sign up for an expedition

All of these milestone goals could be actioned immediately and can be measured day-to-day. Hitting these will, in turn, lead you to complete your overall goal.

Case study

Sarah and Julie both wanted to eat healthier.

Sarah set a goal of "eat healthier at least three times per week". It seemed like a SMART goal as she knew what she wanted to do, how she would measure it and on what timescale.

However, the plan was hard to follow. Sarah could not decide what days to do it on, and when she did make a decision, she spent the whole day searching the internet for recipes that she liked.

Julie set a similar goal. However, she put in more concrete action points. Her goal was "buy a healthy a cookbook, and plan three healthy meals for the week every Sunday".

This approach made executing the plan a lot easier. There were clear steps: buy a cookbook, plan the meals on Sunday, cook the meals on their assigned days. There was no "I'll do that later" or "I'm not sure what to do now" that can lead us to paralyse ourselves with indecision.

Write your goals down

Studies show that you are more likely to follow through on a goal if it is in written form34. Why does writing your plan down help? There are several reasons.

- Written goals are clear. There is no ambiguity. You can review the SMART criteria against what you have written and see if it matches up.
- Written goals are fixed. It is easy for a goal that only exists in your mind to experience scope creep or subtle changes. Exercise three times a week becomes "exercise 2-3 times a week". You went twice last

34 John Traugott. Achieving your goals: An evidence-based approach. Michigan State University. 26 August 2014.
http://msue.anr.msu.edu/news/achieving_your_goals_an_evidence_based_approach

week, so you've hit that goal, right? It is easy to sell ourselves this story. It is a lot harder when we have it written down35.

- The process of writing helps you think the problem through. What are you looking to achieve? Articulating in on paper helps you clarify the goal you are focusing in on.
- Writing it down makes it more real. I talk a lot about behaviours, rather than thoughts. Writing a goal down is a behaviour. It is you committing to a goal. Not just in your mind, but by using behaviour.

Writing down your goals, which is not a massive exercise in itself, can make you nearly twice as likely to follow through with them36.

Goal-setting summary

When people set poor goals, they fail to achieve them. When people set better goals, they are far more likely to succeed. If you have failed in the past, it was almost probably because it was a badly-set goal. Spending time setting better goals will help us achieve them.

Graded exposure

"How do you eat an elephant? One bite at a time." Creighton Abrams

In anxiety therapy, we use a technique called graded exposure. When we exposure ourselves to anxiety, we break it down into a small, manageable steps which are easy to complete. You can repeat each step as many times as you like until it becomes easier, before moving on to the next step.

We do this because if we tried to do everything at once, we would become overwhelmed and give up. This situation is just like when we try to make multiple changes at once.

We can only really concentrate on one thing at a time, so for a complex task, we need to break it down. When I am learning piano, my piano teacher never has me "just play" a brand new piece.

---

35 Robert B. Cialdini. Influence: The Psychology of Persuasion. 26 December 2006. ISBN: 006124189X

36 Dr. Gail Matthews. Goals Research Summary. Dominican University. 9 January 2017. http://www.dominican.edu/academics/ahss/undergraduate-programs/psych/faculty/assets-gail-matthews/researchsummary2.pdf

First, he has me play the notes for the right hand. Just the right hand. Then we do the left hand on its own. After that, we put both hands together, getting the notes in the correct order. After that we do it at the proper tempo. Then we look at dynamics. Each step is isolated and done individually, gradually building up.

We want to do the same thing here. Whenever we want to make a change, we should ask ourselves "can I break this down into more manageable steps?"

If the steps are easy, then great, we can fly through them. However, if they turn out to be harder than we imagined, which is possible once you add anxiety into the mix, we can stop and repeat a step until we feel comfortable with it.

How does this work in the context of lifestyle? Let's say we have decided to eat healthier and cook more at home. Here are five ways you could make the first step a smaller one and then build up to something bigger:

- Start by cooking one night a week, and then build up to more days
- Start by cooking simple meals, then build up to complex ones
- Start by replacing your snacks with healthier alternatives
- Start by making healthier choices for your drinks
- Stop skipping breakfast on weekends, then gradually introduce it to weekdays too

Similarly, if you want to exercise more, maybe there is one journey you can identify that you will walk from now on.

Increasing motivation

Once we have set our goals, how to we make sure that we follow through on them? In this section, we will review options for increasing our motivation.

Using easy goals to build up wins

During the Q&A session of a talk I was delivering, someone once asked me what I thought of New Year's Resolutions. I told them this: "set yourself a target of going to the gym three times per year".

Sounds crazy, right? The person who asked the question was almost certainly saying to themselves "three times per year? I want to be going every week!"

But I stand by my answer. Why? Because people do not stick to their resolutions. In one study, only 19% of dieters managed to keep theirs[37]. In fact, many of us consider the whole thing a joke because we know that we never stick to them.

This mindset is harmful because it sets us up for failure. We teach ourselves that we are not people who achieve our goals[38]. Subconsciously we tell ourselves that we will not follow through.

So, back to my gym example. Set a resolution to go three times per year. You can hit that. At the end of the year, you will have over-delivered on it. Then double your goal. In year two, have an objective of going six times. It's just three *extra* times, right?

What happens if you keep doing this?

Year	Gym visits
Year 1	3 visits
Year 2	6 visits
Year 3	12 visits
Year 4	24 visits
Year 5	48 visits

By year five, you are going to the gym once a week. And all you have done is hit easy goals and increased your target each year by no more than you were doing already.

You are probably thinking "five years? I can't wait that long." You're right; it is a long time. But how long have you waited already? Most people spend decades going in and out of gym routines. Year after year setting a new resolution and then failing to meet it. We have *already* waited too long to make these changes. So, this time, let's do it in a way that works.

In this book, we won't be waiting five years for results. However, I wanted you to understand the importance of the feedback cycle. We need to train ourselves that we are people who achieve our goals.

---

37 Norcross JC, Vangarelli DJ. The resolution solution: longitudinal examination of New Year's change attempts. J Subst Abuse. 1988-1989;1(2):127-34.

38 NHS Choices. 10 tips to make your New Year's resolution a success. 18 December 2016. http://www.nhs.uk/Livewell/Healthychristmas/Pages/NewYearresolutions.aspx

We will be using a shorter feedback cycle. However, it is okay to start off slow and build up. In fact, it was way better and will produce far more results in the long term. Set easy goals at first, teach your brain that you are someone who completes them, and then make them more difficult.

Essentially, this is a reversal of the change resistance cycle. Each little task we succeed at gives us positive feedback that we can make a change, and therefore provides us with more motivation for the next one.

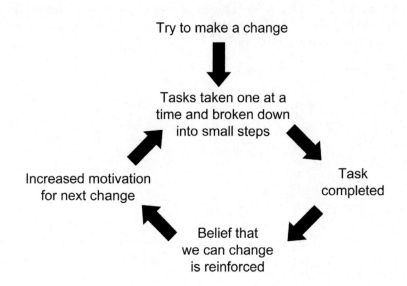

Temptation bundling

Battling against your desire to stay on the sofa is always going to be an uphill battle. You have to wrestle with yourself every week. Sometimes you will win, sometimes you will lose. It is not a perfect system.

But what if you could make yourself *want* to go out and exercise? What if you could find a way to be excited about exercising? How much easier would that be? The answer is a lot. But how exactly can we do that?

Three researchers: Katherine Milkman, Julia Minson and Kevin Volpp, may have the answer. In a paper titled ***Holding The Hunger Games***

Hostage at the Gym: An Evaluation of Temptation Bundling39 they describe a technique known as "temptation bundling" that could have just that effect.

The idea is that you restrict something you want to do so that it is only permissible when doing something you want to motivate yourself to do. In the research paper, they looked at exercise.

They provided test subjects with some iPods pre-loaded with a selection of tempting audiobooks. The control group were told they could listen whenever they wanted. The treatment group were told that the iPods had to be kept at the gym, and could only be used while they were exercising.

The result? Those who could only continue their novel by going to the gym went to the gym more often. People were more motivated when there was a temptation bundled in.

Here is how Milkman described it in her own words on the Freakonomics podcast40.

"So what if you only let yourself get a pedicure while catching up on overdue emails for work? Or what if you only let yourself listen to your favourite CDs while catching up on household chores. Or only let yourself go to your very favourite restaurant whose hamburgers you crave while spending time with a difficult relative who you should see more of."

We do not have a team of gym staff and scientists to keep an eye on us (not that they were checking up on people that much in the research, but the social pressure was there), but with some self-restraint, we may be able to implement similar systems ourselves.

Here are some possible suggestions for how temptation bundling can be used in a variety of situations:

Temptation	But only when...
Listening to your favourite music	Going for a run

39 Katherine L. Milkman, Julia A. Minson, Kevin G. M. Volpp. Holding the Hunger Games Hostage at the Gym: An Evaluation of Temptation Bundling. Management Science 201460:2, 283-299. DOI: http://dx.doi.org/10.1287/mnsc.2013.1784

40 Stephen J. Dubner. When Willpower Isn't Enough. Freakonomics Radio. 13 March 2015.

Playing games on your tablet	You are out in the fresh air
Wearing your favourite outfit	You are in challenging social situations
Checking Facebook	At the library studying

Getting support from others

Friends, family and the wider society can play a critical role in helping us achieve our goals.

Should we announce our goals?

The evidence for publicly announcing your goals is mixed. Robert Cialdini argues that you should41. Publicly announcing your goals has some advantages:

1. You want people to think highly of you, and will, therefore, be more motivated not to let them down.
2. A public declaration engages our need to be consistent with what we say, and therefore creates psychological pressure to follow through.

However, Derek Sivers argues that you should keep your goals to yourself. For example, just announcing to all of your friends that you are on a new diet or starting a new exercise routine may be a bad idea42.

This is because, in the act of telling them, and usually them congratulating you, you receive some of the gratification immediately, even though you have not done anything yet. This makes you less likely to complete the goal43 because you feel like you are already half way there (even though you haven't started).

If you do decide to announce your goals in advance, you need to consider the method that you do it: it needs to be clear what your goal is and that you want people to hold you accountable, rather than congratulate you in advance.

---

41 Robert B. Cialdini. Influence: The Psychology of Persuasion. 26 December 2006. ISBN: 006124189X

42 Peter M. Gollwitzer, Paschal Sheeran, Verena Michalski, and Andrea E. Seifert. When Intentions Go Public: Does Social Reality Widen the Intention-Behavior Gap? Psychological Science May 2009 vol. 20 no. 5 612-618. DOI: 10.1111/j.1467-9280.2009.02336.x

43 Derek Sivers. Keep your goals to yourself. TEDGlobal 2010.

Report results, not intentions

If we decide to keep our goals private, we want to ensure we get the gratification once we have done something. We can collect praise and support for the things that we **have** done.

Therefore, when you do achieve something, that is the time to share it with your friends.

Put your goals in a wider context

When writing your goals, you can consider how they will affect the people close to you. For example, if your goal was to spend more time with your family, don't just write:

"I want to spend more time with my family."

Instead, write:

"I want to spend more time with my family as they enjoy seeing me."

Putting your goals in a wider context, and giving it meaning beyond your personal benefit, makes you more likely to follow through44.

Get a gym buddy

You are far more likely to stay motivated if you have someone to do it with. This effect is not just confined to the gym: any form of exercise benefits from a social dynamic45.

When you undertake exercise with someone else, you feel motivated not to let them down. This feeling makes it easier to turn up: there is a feeling of social responsibility. It also creates a positive role model to inspire you. All

---

44 Fitzsimons, G. M., & Finkel, E. J. (2010). Interpersonal influences on self regulation. Current Directions in Psychological Science, 19, 101-105.

45 Homa Khaleeli, Bella Mackie, John Crace. Staying healthy: why a fitness buddy is all you need. The Guardian. 23 April 2016.
https://www.theguardian.com/lifeandstyle/2016/apr/23/fitness-buddies-exercise-boxing-running-gym-with-friends

of this leads to you working harder when you are exercising with people you like46.

Exercising in a larger group is also beneficial: it creates social bonds between the group that inspire you to perform better47.

The same technique can be applied to any area, not just exercise. One of my friends used to have a fruit and veg competition with her partner. Rather than aiming for the classic "5 portions a day", they would outdo each other trying to find new and unique vegetables to eat.

Make commitment contracts

We are motivated by gains, but even more motivated by loss aversion. That is to say: we will work hard to avoid losing something48.

How can we leverage this in a social motivation context?

Give your friend £100 and tell them not to give it back unless you complete a specific goal. Have them burn the money or give it away to a charity you hate: you need to feel the pain of loss to get maximum motivation.

Note that they should not give the money to a charity you like. Doing this provides a get-out: you can tell yourself that failing is a good thing because a charity is benefiting. It needs to hurt.

Such contracts can be arranged online via websites such as stickK49.

Using the power of habit

One of the reasons people begin something and then give up is that they do not make it a habit. Change takes a certain amount of effort, whereas habit takes much less.

---

46 Brandon Irwin. Motivational losing: being the weak link in team activities may lead to longer, more intense workouts. Kansas State University. 26 November 2012. https://www.k-state.edu/media/newsreleases/nov12/exercise112612.html

47 Davis A, Taylor J, Cohen E (2015) Social Bonds and Exercise: Evidence for a Reciprocal Relationship. PLoS ONE 10(8): e0136705. doi:10.1371/journal.pone.0136705

48 Daniel Kahneman. Thinking, Fast and Slow. 25 October 2011. ISBN: 0374275637

49 stickK, http://www.stickk.com/

This means that when you begin making a change, it takes a lot of effort. You have to think about doing it consciously. This is fine because when you start something you often have the highest level of motivation to do it, so you are fired up. However, as time goes by that motivation decreases. By the time it does, we want to have the change as a habit.

Habits are much easier to follow because they do not place the same cognitive load on our brains. We just do them. Think about driving, for example. For most people who can drive, it is pretty easy. You have practised it until you can do it without thinking about it. We are aiming for the same thing here; we want the behaviour to be automatic.

Failing to turn a change into a habit will result in failure once we lose our initial motivation.

Let's look at an example. Say we want to start going for a run once a week. We need to make this a habit. We do this by assigning a specific day and time when we go for a run. This could be anything, but we will pick noon on Sundays for this example.

Once you set this time, and start doing it, you have a habit. Your brain knows that when it gets to noon on Sunday, you go for a run. That is what you do. There is nothing to think about: it is running time.

In contrast, what would happen if you did not set this time? We tell ourselves that we will "just fit it in somewhere". Each day we wonder whether today is the day we should "fit it in". But we do not feel like going for a run today. So we say to ourselves "I will go tomorrow instead". And we do this every day until we have not gone for a run all week.

In the first scenario, we did not feel like going for a run either. However, it did not matter we did not feel like going for a run on Sunday. That was our running time, so we went anyway. There was no decision to make. The cognitive load is reduced, and our habit sticks.

This system is not 100% perfect. Sometimes we will put it off anyway. However, it is far more effective than the second scenario.

How habit driven are we?

One interesting thing I noticed about these habits happened when my daughter was born. When a new baby arrives, the world is turned on its head. Day and night do not seem to have much meaning anymore; you are sleeping when the baby is sleeping and feeding or changing her when she is awake.

What happened to my teeth brushing when my regular daily schedule was up-ended? It still happened, but only on about a 50% success rate. When I had some sense of normality, I would get up and brush my teeth. But on days when she had cried all night, there was not a concept of "morning" in the Worfolk household, so these things were forgotten.

Luckily this only lasted a few weeks until she began to get a sense of night and day. However, the effect it had on my good behaviours did not go unnoticed.

Summary

In this chapter, we looked at some of the techniques we can use to follow through on our goals.

We reminded ourselves that change is hard and that we need to prepare ourselves for the *inevitable* resistance we will experience. We learnt how to make goals more achievable by setting better ones and what systems we can put in place to make sure we follow through with them.

In the next chapter, we will look at how to implement these techniques into a system that will allow us to make sustainable changes to our lifestyle.

The Design-a-lifestyle process

So far we have learnt that using lifestyle changes to manage anxiety is an effective and enjoyable way to manage anxiety because of both the short-term health benefits and the long-term reduction in anxiety.

But how do we go about implementing such changes? In this chapter, we will look at the process step-by-step.

This chapter is **the magic** if you will. It is the system that we will be using to make the changes in our lives.

The system

Here are the six steps:

1. Select a factor of your lifestyle you want to address
2. Select one change to make in this area
3. Create a written plan with SMART goals
4. Execute the plan for at least four weeks
5. Review the results
6. Repeat the process

1. Select a factor

The first thing we need to do is narrow down to an area, or **factor**, that we are going to work on.

What factors will we look at?

There are many different factors that we could consider when looking at lifestyle. In this book, I am going to concentrate on the seven I think are most important. These are exercise, diet, sleep, personal growth, relaxation, relationships and community.

We can plot them on a diagram and use this to measure our progress.

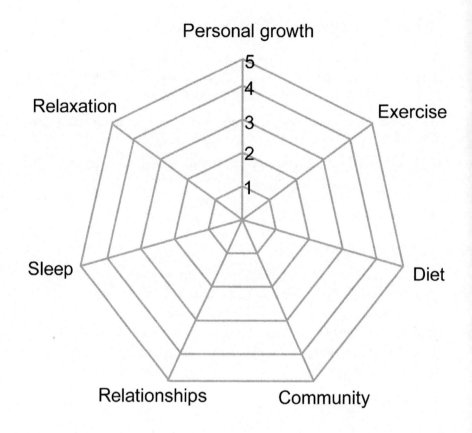

Scoring yourself

If you want an overview of how you are doing at the moment and where you could improve, you can fill out the diagram. This is a personal exercise. To assist you, I have provided some general guidelines below. You will need to apply these to your circumstances.

The suggestions are brief: more context will be added in later chapters as we go through each factor and discuss the different ways we can measure and improve each.

Factor	Signs there could be room to improve	Signs you are scoring highly already
Exercise	Not exercising, or if you do, only occasionally and	Having a regular exercise programme that

	infrequently.	you stick to.
Diet	Being over or under weight. Not having a rough idea of your weight and target BMI. Skipping meals. Regularly eating fast food. Eating unhealthy food. Using fad diets. Drinking excessively. Smoking.	Eating healthy meals. Planning meals. Limiting fast food, processed and red meat. Cooking. Being in control of your weight. Being in control of your drinking. Staying hydrated.
Sleep	Sleeping less than seven or more than nine hours per night. Being unable to fall asleep or stay asleep. Irregular sleep patterns. Using sleeping tablets.	Sleeping 7-9 hours per night. Having a routine and bedtime. Designing your sleeping environment and removing distractions. Being kind to yourself during bouts of insomnia.
Relaxation	Not allowing yourself to relax. Not enjoying your relaxation time.	Investing in relaxation time, doing an activity you enjoy. Being kind to yourself.
Personal growth	Not undertaking any personal growth or learning. Not having a regular schedule.	Being on a course. Learning something new, ideally on a schedule. Working towards a goal.
Relationships	Having less than three close relationships. Irregular social contact.	Regular social contact with family and friends. Being able to be open with people close to you. Being able to talk about anxiety with others. Using gratitude techniques.
Community	Not being involved in any community groups.	Regularly attending community groups. Taking a leadership role in a group. Holding down a job.

2. Select one change to make

Once we know what we want to focus on, we need to select one change to make in our lives. At this point, we can stay general: in the next step, we will get very specific about what we want to do.

Here are some examples:

Factor	Change
Exercise	Join a gym and go once per week.
Diet	Eat vegetarian meals on Saturdays.
Relationships	See my friends at least twice per week.

Why stick to one change at a time

We only have so much attention and so much motivation. Willpower is a finite resource50. Therefore, it is important to direct this energy into mastering one thing at a time.

If not, we quickly become overwhelmed, tell ourselves that we cannot do it, and give up. To avoid this, we need to make each change on its own.

We are looking to build habits here. We want each change to be incorporated into our everyday life without having to think about it. Making a change takes a lot of willpower; continuing a habit does not.

We should not move on until we have mastered the change and made it part of our everyday life. If we try to do two things at once, our energy will be divided, and we will be less likely to succeed. Taking each change in isolation is slower, but builds up lasting results.

Case study

Cheryl was determined to start exercising every day and cooking a healthy meal every night. This was a big ask given she already worked full time.

For the first week, everything went well. Then she started to run out of time. She found that she had to pick between using the two hours she had to exercise or to cook.

---

50 Baumeister, et al. (1998). Ego depletion: is the active self a limited resource? Journal of Personality and Social Psychology, 74, 1252-1265.

She made different choices on different days. All of a sudden she was not somebody who exercises every day, nor someone who eats healthily every day. It then became too easy not to do either of them when she was busy because neither was a daily habit.

Sticking to just one would have allowed her to dedicate all of her time and energy to getting that down to a habit. This approach gives her more chance to keep it up and feel better about herself.

Selecting a change

When selecting a change, should you attack your weaknesses or play to your strengths?

The traditional view is that you should focus on improving your weaknesses. This is the view I most recommend as it allows you to make the most amount of improvement.

There is an old rule of thumb called the 80/20 rule. This says that you can achieve 80% of the result with 20% of the effort while getting the remaining 20% of the result takes 80% of the effort. Consider world-class athletes, for example. It is relatively easy to become **quite good** at a sport, but to be world-class takes a lifetime of dedication.

Therefore, if we want to make the most improvement, we should pick something we are not doing that well at because relatively little effort should produce significant results.

However, there is a counter argument to this, one that I have previously written about[51]. The problem with focusing on your weaknesses is that it is hard to motivate yourself to do something you do not like.

Typically, your strengths will be your strengths because you enjoy them and spend time working on them, while your weaknesses will be there because you do not enjoy them and do not want to spend time on them. Therefore, it is easier to find the motivation to work on your strengths.

---

51 Chris Worfolk. Thinking about New Year's resolutions? Read this first. http://blog.chrisworfolk.com/2015/12/31/thinking-about-new-years-resolutions-read-this-first/

Do not get hung up

When it comes to making a choice, do not hang around too long. You do not need to make a perfect choice; you just need to choose something that is **good enough**.

Why do I say this? It is easy to get wrapped up in not knowing what to change, and finding yourself paralysed by indecision and not making any change.

Barry Schwartz sums this up in his book The Paradox of Choice52. If we aim to be perfectionists in our decision making, we end up spending too much time on them, driving ourselves crazy trying to weight up every single fact and then worrying we have made the incorrect choice after we have done it. Whereas if we just make a **good enough** choice and get on with it, we are happier and more productive.

Do not worry if the change you choose to make seems imperfect. As long as it is one that you are somewhat excited about making, it will be good enough.

Case study

Darren wanted to make a change. He went over and over in his mind as to what would be the best one to make. He realised that he had spent two weeks trying to decide on the perfect change, and yet had not done anything yet.

Instead, he decided to accept that his first decision may not be the optimal one, picked one and went with it. This way he had done the most important thing: taking action.

The truth is, it does not matter if you make a **wrong** choice. You are starting in the process of making changes and following through on them. That in itself is valuable.

3. Create a written plan

We now know what we want to do. The next step is to translate this into a set of goals and actionable steps. To make sure our memory does not play games with us, we need to write this down as a written plan.

---

52 Barry Schwartz. The Paradox of Choice: Why More Is Less. 18 January 2005. ISBN: 0060005696

Here is an example of a poorly written plan:

"Go for runs all the time."

This goal is not specific or measurable. What exactly is ***all the time***? How will we know if we succeed? Compare that to the example below, which is much better:

"Go running once a week on a Saturday morning. Exercise for at least half an hour. Post results to friends on Strava. Only listen to my new audiobook during this time."

This goal is much better. It is simple to measure success. It creates a habit: Saturday mornings are running mornings. It has a social component and includes temptation bundling.

Here is another bad example:

"Become vegetarian."

This goal is not very actionable: where do you start? If you are a meat eater, cutting out meat altogether is probably too large a step to stick to all at once. Here is a better example:

"Buy a vegetarian cookbook and introduce meat-free dinners on Monday evenings. Share pictures of the meals I make with my friends on Instagram."

This one has clear action steps, does not require huge changes and includes a social component.

It takes practice to write high-quality goals. I often have to revise my first draft. Here is a checklist for everything you should consider. You do not need to hit everything with each goal, but the more, the better.

Is my goal a SMART goal?

- [ ] Is the goal specific?
- [ ] Is it clear how you can measure your progress?
- [ ] Is it achievable?
- [ ] Are there clear time constraints?

Actions

- [ ] Are there clear action steps?
- [ ] Does it break it down into small enough steps?

- [] How will this become a habit in the long term?

Influences

- [] Have you considered a social component?
- [] Have you considered a commitment contract?
- [] Have you considered temptation bundling?

4. Execute the plan

Your goal is written down, and it looks awesome. Finally, we can dispense with the paperwork and do something! It is time to execute your plan.

How long do I need to do it for?

As long as you want, but at least four weeks. We want to do it until it becomes habit. There are some factors that can influence this:

- How often you do it. If your goal is "eat breakfast three times per week" you will have bigger sample size after four weeks than you will if your goal is "run once per week".
- How easy you find it to develop new habits.

It takes a long time to build a habit. In 2010, University College London (UCL) published a study53 showing just how long it requires. The results: it took **18 to 254 days** for people to turn their new behaviour into a habit. A second paper, published by the same team54, showed the *average* time was **66 days**.

Typically, it takes at least two months to bed in a habit. However, we want to review our progress before that point, so 28 days makes a sensible point to do that.

---

53 Lally, P., van Jaarsveld, C. H. M., Potts, H. W. W. and Wardle, J. (2010), How are habits formed: Modelling habit formation in the real world. Eur. J. Soc. Psychol., 40: 998–1009. doi:10.1002/ejsp.674

54 Benjamin Gardner, Phillippa Lally, Jane Wardle. Making health habitual: the psychology of 'habit-formation' and general practice. Br J Gen Pract. 2012 Dec; 62(605): 664–666. DOI: doi: 10.3399/bjgp12X659466

Write down your results

When discussing writing down our plan, we looked at why it was important: our memory lies to us and misleads us. The same thing applies to results. We need to record our results, tracking real numbers. Be specific.

Below, I have outlined some examples of questions we need to ask ourselves.

Factor	Task	What to record
Exercise	Work out for 30 minutes.	How long did you actually work out for? Not the time you got to the gym, or left the gym: actual work out time.
Sleep	Go to bed at 11 pm	What time did you actually go to bed? What time did you stop playing with your phone?
Personal growth	Do more reading	How long did you read for? Technically, reading for two minutes is reading every day, but not very productive.

5. Review the results

After four weeks, it is time to review your results. How well did you do? Review your written records and see how often you hit your goal.

Depending on how well you did, will depend on what you should do next.

If you consistently missed your goal, do not beat yourself up. It was a poorly designed goal. Review your plan, and adjust it to make it easier. Then execute it again.

If you consistently hit your goal and you feel comfortable with it, consider making it at little harder for the next four weeks. Instead of going out of the house two times a week, set it to three times per week.

If you consistently hit your goal but do not feel comfortable, just keep executing the plan for another for weeks. There is no rush. Remember that it can take 2-8 months to build a habit.

If you have already completed the cycle several times, you may feel comfortable that it is a habit now. If most of the resistance to doing the task has disappeared (not all of it needs to go, and probably never will), congratulations, you have indeed formed a new habit! It is time to pick an entirely new goal and move on.

6. Repeat the process

You're done: you have made it through the entire cycle! You are now ready to go back to the start and make another change to your lifestyle.

Summary

That is it: the whole process. Remember that the system is simple in principle, but hard to follow through on. It takes practice and deliberate effort.

In the following chapters, we will look at each lifestyle factor in turn. We will review what the evidence says for each, and how we can make improvements.

Exercise

Exercise is a great place to start because it is often considered "the thing" to do when you are trying to lead a healthier lifestyle.

This is unfair on the other factors, which are equally important. However, exercise is certainly a cornerstone of healthy living. It also makes an excellent topic of focus because we know how much exercise is needed and it is easy to track how much you are doing.

The benefits of exercise

Exercise produces a broad range of advantages. It helps both your physical and your mental health. It also produces pleasurable feelings and gets you outside the house.

Physical benefits of exercise

Exercise improves your overall health. There is a correlation between physical and mental health. Therefore, if your body is healthier, you will feel better, have more energy and are more likely to experience higher mood.

Exercise makes it easier to fight off infection[55]. This means you are less likely to get a cold, and that it will be less severe when you do get one. This goes for other diseases too. Less illness is likely to increase your mood, especially if you have health anxiety and worry about becoming ill.

Mental benefits of exercise

Exercise helps with mood stability[56]. This effect is true for everyone but is particularly the case for people with anxiety and depression, who experience the greatest uplift. It makes you feel less tired, less angry and less tense.

---

55 Harvard Health Publications, "How to boost your immune system", http://www.health.harvard.edu/staying-healthy/how-to-boost-your-immune-system

56 Lane AM1, Lovejoy DJ. The effects of exercise on mood changes: the moderating effect of depressed mood. J Sports Med Phys Fitness. 2001 Dec;41(4):539-45.

Exercise improves your ability to handle stress57. It does this by releasing short bursts of cortisol, sometimes called the "stress hormone", and your body then adapts to cope with this. When you stop exercising, your cortisol levels go back to normal, but your body remembers the lesson and handles stress better in the future.

Exercise gives you something else to think about. Distraction is a tactic often used by anxiety sufferers to take their mind off their anxiety. Exercise turns out to be an excellent way of distracting yourself.58.

Feel the (mental pain)

Exercise induces similar symptoms to anxiety and panic attacks. You find yourself short of breath, your heart racing, your chest being tight and maybe even a little dizzy.

Some people find this is a useful exercise in itself. You learn that these symptoms are not harmful to you in the long term and have the chance to see them in a positive light.

Runner's high

The term *runner's high* is not restricted to running, but rather describes the feeling you experience when undertaking prolonged intense exercise.

It is a measurable phenomenon and is not just found to humans59. Other mammals, including dogs, seem to experience the same thing.

How effective is exercise?

Very effective. A Cochrane Review of exercise found that it was just as good as any drug or therapy for dealing with depression60.

---

57 Wikipedia, Neurobiological effects of physical exercise". 28 October 2016. https://en.wikipedia.org/wiki/Neurobiological_effects_of_physical_exercise

58 Zschucke E, Gaudlitz K, Ströhle A. Exercise and Physical Activity in Mental Disorders: Clinical and Experimental Evidence. Journal of Preventive Medicine and Public Health. 2013;46(Suppl 1):S12-S21. doi:10.3961/jpmph.2013.46.S.S12.

59 David A. Raichlen, Adam D. Foster, Gregory L. Gerdeman, Alexandre Seillier, Andrea Giuffrida. Wired to run: exercise-induced endocannabinoid signaling in humans and cursorial mammals with implications for the 'runner's high'. Journal of Experimental Biology 2012 215: 1331-1336; doi: 10.1242/jeb.063677

Going outside

An added benefit of going outside and exercising is the *going outside* bit. This alone is beneficial for a number of reasons.

Getting some sun

Telling you that you need to go outside to get some sun on your face sounds patronising. Also, if you, like myself, live in the UK, you are probably more likely to be standing under a cloud than any direct sunlight even if you do go out.

However, research shows that it is important[61]. The primary benefit of getting some sun is it boosts your body's vitamin D supply, which provides an overall benefit for your health. It may also help:

* Prevent autoimmune disease
* Reduce cancer risk
* Improve skin conditions

You do not need to be outside long to get enough exposure. 5-30 minutes between 10 am and 3 pm twice a week is sufficient[62].

Engaging with nature

Reconnecting with nature sounds like a phrase touted by hippies. It is. However, research has shown that spending more time in a natural environment, opposed to an urbanised one, could make us feel better.

A study by Stanford University looked at participants who were sent on a 90-minute walk through a natural environment. They found that the participants who did the walk had calmer minds and were less anxious[63].

---

60 Cooney GM, Dwan K, Greig CA, Lawlor DA, Rimer J, Waugh FR, McMurdo M, Mead GE. Exercise for depression. Cochrane Database of Systematic Reviews 2013, Issue 9. Art. No.: CD004366. DOI: 10.1002/14651858.CD004366.pub6.

61 M. Nathaniel Mead. Benefits of Sunlight: A Bright Spot for Human Health. Environ Health Perspect. 2008 Apr; 116(4): A160–A167.

62 Ising H, Kruppa B. Health effects caused by noise: Evidence in the literature from the past 25 years. Noise Health 2004;6:5-13

Smell those smells

If reconnecting with nature was not hippie enough, wait until I tell you that certain smells *could* help.

A 2010 study suggested that jasmine could uplift your mood64. It was published in a journal named ***Natural product communications***. This does not sound that credible, but their journal impact factor is inline with others65. Other sources point out that evidence is limited66.

How much exercise do I need to do?

NHS guidelines suggest that you should do at least two and a half hours of moderate activity per week or 75 minutes of vigorous activity per week67. This differs slightly for children and elderly people.

Moderate activity includes:

- Power walking
- Gentle swimming
- Hiking
- Cycling
- Low-intensity sports

It should leave you a little out of breath, and warm you up a little, but you should still be able to talk.

Vigorous activity includes:

- Running

---

63 Gregory N. Bratman, J. Paul Hamilton, Kevin S. Hahn, Gretchen C. Daily, and James J. Gross. Nature experience reduces rumination and subgenual prefrontal cortex activation. PNAS. 14 July 14 2015 vol. 112 no. 28. DOI: 10.1073/pnas.1510459112

64 Hongratanaworakit T. Stimulating effect of aromatherapy massage with jasmine oil. Nat Prod Commun. 2010 Jan;5(1):157-62.

65 Natural product communications Journal Impact. ResearchGate. 28 October 2016. https://www.researchgate.net/journal/1934-578X_Natural_product_communications

66 Critical Cactus. Do Aromatherapy Scents At Home Really Make You Feel Better? 10 February 2014. http://www.criticalcactus.com/aromatherapy-scents-home/

67 NHS Choices, "Physical activity guidelines for adults", http://www.nhs.uk/Livewell/fitness/Pages/physical-activity-guidelines-for-adults.aspx

- Fast swimming
- Cycling up hills
- Most team sports
- Martial arts

Vigorous activity should noticeably raise your heart rate, leave you out of breath to the point that it makes it difficult to talk and causes you to sweat.

This amount reflects guidelines for staying physically healthy. The exact amount required to keep your mind healthy is more open to interpretation. In Michael Otto and Jasper A.J. Smits' book *Exercise for Mood and Anxiety*, they come up with the following suggestion[68].

"500 to 1,000 metabolic equivalency tasks (METs) minutes per week."

A metabolic equivalency task (MET) is a system to allow you to compare different levels of exercise intensity. To draw a parallel with the NHS guidelines above, moderate exercise would be worth around 5 METs and vigorous exercise would be worth around 10 METs.

Therefore, if we translate that into time we get:

Intensity of exercise	Time per week
Moderate	100-200 minutes (2-3 hours)
Vigorous	50-100 minutes (1-2 hours)

These guidelines is roughly inline with the guidelines for staying physically healthy.

What exercise should I do?

Anything you like! Ideally, you will pick something you enjoy as that will make it easier to motivate yourself. Accessibility is an important consideration too, though. Skiing might be a lot of fun, but it is hard to do it several times a week!

---

68 Michael Otto Ph.D., Jasper A.J. Smits Ph.D. Exercise for Mood and Anxiety: Proven Strategies for Overcoming Depression and Enhancing Well-Being. 28 July 2011. ISBN: 0199791007

Walking

Walking is a highly accessible form of exercise. You can do it pretty much anywhere, you do not need any special equipment, and your level of fitness is irrelevant because you can start at any level.

Often you do not even need to schedule additional time for walking. You can switch your commute to work or other travels to walking. Walking to work and back every day will probably fill your recommended exercise quota for the week.

Even if you do not have a walkable commute, or do not have any commute at all, walking can still be put into the context of being useful. You could walk to the shops every day to buy some bread and milk, for example. Even if you do a weekly shop, you could motivate yourself by leaving out a few key items that you will walk to the shops for during the week.

Doing this may feel like a waste of time at first: why would you deliberately leave out items to create work for yourself? The answer is that the goal is motivating you to exercise. Having to buy milk will provide that.

As you progress, walking can expand too. You can increase your distances, or travel to the countryside and take in a particular route or scenic walk. There are plenty of walking groups too, including groups for retired and unemployed people that take place during working hours.

Running

Running is another accessible option. You can run anywhere, and you do not need any special equipment, other than perhaps a pair of trainers and jogging bottoms. That is not to say you cannot get plenty of gear: I have a GPS device, leggings, running shoes, the list goes on. But I do not **need** any of this stuff to go running.

I also like it because it has a high exercise to time spent ratio. If I go to the gym or the swimming pool I spent more time in the logistics than I do exercising. I have to travel to the gym, get changed, do the exercise, have a shower, wash my hair, get changed and go home. With running, I can set off from my front door and the only real non-exercise time spent is the shower I have when I get home (which I would probably have anyway).

There are lots of easy ways to get into running.

I like Parkrun69. It is a free 5km run that takes place at 9 am every Saturday morning in most parks in the UK, and increasingly across the world as well.

Here is how it works: you register online and are given a unique barcode to print out. You then turn up and do the actual run itself. Sizes vary with a few dozen people at smaller runs to a few hundred people at larger ones. When you finish the run, a marshal will scan your barcode, and this records your time.

It has particular appeal to me as a Yorkshireman, as there are prizes for completing a set number of runs. At 50, 100 and 250 runs, you receive a free t-shirt (though you do have to pay for delivery).

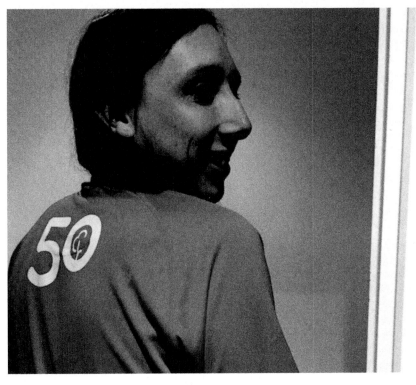

Another great option is the Couch to 5k (C25K) programme70. C25K is a programme specifically designed for someone who has never run before,

69 Parkrun, http://www.parkrun.org.uk/

70 Couch to 5K, http://www.nhs.uk/Livewell/c25k/Pages/couch-to-5k.aspx

taking them from not being a runner to being able to run 5km or at least 30 minutes, over a period of nine weeks.

Here is how it works: you download the app to your phone, and it provides you with guided workouts. There are three per week, each lasting for 30 minutes. It starts with a gentle run-a-bit walk-a-bit phase and builds up. The app integrates with your music apps so that you can listen to your music while working out. It is free, or you can pay to remove the adverts.

Swimming

Swimming is highly beneficial exercise[71], as well as being very pleasurable. Therefore, even though it can be a hassle to travel to the pool and back, you may consider that that is time well invested.

If you are lucky, the pool might also have a sauna, steam room or hot tub as well. I found that the combination of a vigorous swim followed by a soak in the hot tub did wonders for my relaxation.

If you are feeling brave, you can then jump back into the pool after being in the sauna. We do this when swimming in lakes in Finland. It makes for a refreshing plunge! Though in fairness, I have never dared try it in winter yet.

---

71 Paul D. Thompson, David Buchner, Ileana L. Piña, Gary J. Balady, Mark A. Williams, Bess H. Marcus, Kathy Berra, Steven N. Blair, Fernando Costa, Barry Franklin, Gerald F. Fletcher, Neil F. Gordon, Russell R. Pate, Beatriz L. Rodriguez, Antronette K. Yancey and Nanette K. Wenger. Exercise and Physical Activity in the Prevention and Treatment of Atherosclerotic Cardiovascular Disease. Circulation. June 24, 2003, Volume 107, Issue 24. DOI: http://dx.doi.org/10.1161/01.CIR.0000075572.40158.77

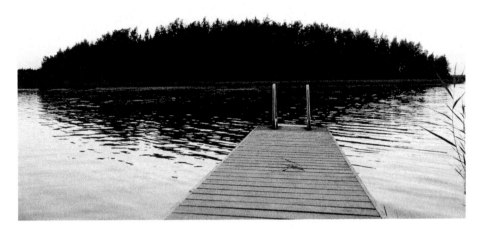

Other sports

Today, the internet makes it very easy to find a local sports club or activity. There is a remarkable range of recognised sports available. In England for example, Sport England recognise 100 different sports, not including the various disciplines within those sports72.

Google, Meetup and Facebook are all common places to find local sports clubs. If you are in the UK, BBC Sport's Get Inspired73 can be very helpful too as you do not need to know what you are looking for before you go searching for it.

If you are stuck for ideas, here are some fun sports you might want to try:

- *Dance*. I think dance is probably one of the most underrated exercises you can do, especially among men. It is an excellent workout and gets you meeting lots of new people. It is hard to get bored of because there are so many different styles. If you are wondering how to get started,

---

72 Sport England. Sporting Activities and Governing Bodies Recognised by the Sports Councils. April 2016.

73 BBC Sport Get Inspired, http://www.bbc.co.uk/sport/get-inspired

try *ceroc*. It is a form of jive that does away with the complicated footwork. There are many local groups that welcome beginners.

- **Badminton**: Given that you are just swatting at a little shuttlecock, it is surprisingly how fast badminton can cause you to break a sweat. It is also pretty easy to set up. You just need a patch of grass or a hall. Of course, a net and a marked-out pitch are nice additions, but my wife and I often just take our £8 racket set to the park and play there.

- **Quidditch**: If you have read **Harry Potter**, which I am guessing you have, you have probably thought to yourself "well, quidditch looks fun, but obviously you cannot do it in the real world". It turns out that they have made a muggle version of it. There is no flying, but there are broomsticks, a quaffle, bludgers and a snitch. There is even a governing body: the International Quidditch Association.

- **Walking football**: A version of regular football where you are not allowed to run. It is aimed at the over 50s, allowing a more leisurely but still competitive version of the game.

- **Taekwondo**: Taekwondo is my favourite martial art because it is all about the kicking. Some martial arts are all about getting up close and personal. They involve getting right in someone's face. Not taekwondo. It is about standing as far away as possible from your opponent and using your longest limb. Not only is it a great workout, but you get a mental workout from learning the patterns, it is perfect for self-discipline and a lot safer than people often imagine.

- **Flag football**: If you have ever watched NFL or any American football, you may have thought to yourself "that looks fun, but I do not fancy getting hurt". It is a fair reason. We have lives to get on with and cannot afford to be going around with broken bones. Luckily, there is an alternative. Flag football is a 5-a-side non-contact version that is more fun, has a faster pace, and involves less standing around and much less injury.

- **Octopush**: This sounds like the most made-up sport ever. That is fine when you remember that all sports are **made-up** at some point in their history. Octopush is underwater hockey. You get a mask and a snorkel, and the puck is on the bottom of the pool. It is as mad as it sounds: look it up on YouTube. Then go out and give it a try.

- **Climbing**: Climbing has become very trendy recently. The increase in the number of indoor climbing walls has made it more accessible. Most centres run beginners courses or taster sessions.

- **Kabaddi**: Okay, I admit that you are probably not going to try this one. But I could not resist slipping it in. **Kabaddi** is a South Asian sport where you have to hold your breath, run into your opponent's half of the court, tag them, and then run back before you run out of oxygen. Their job is to wrestle you to the ground and prevent you from getting back to your half. How does the referee know you are holding your breath? You have to chant "kabaddi" the whole time. It is a fun game to watch.

Are martial arts safe?

Some people may worry about getting hurt while doing martial arts. I must admit that when I started, I was concerned too. Anything where you have to put pads on, suggests that you have them for a reason.

However, my experience of taekwondo has been a safe one. I have never seen a serious injury. The worst I have seen was when one of my friends accidentally caught another of my friends in the groin. I felt his pain that day, but he managed to run it off.

This safety is not my experience with other sports. Football, which is not supposed to be a high contract sport, has sent many of my friends to the hospital. There is some risk when you do any sport of course, but martial arts do not seem to be particularly hazardous.

Team sports

I will discuss team sports in more detail in the section on community. Team sports are a double win because it gives you a chance to build new relationships while exercising at the same time.

Finding time for exercise

Exercise is very time-consuming. If we assume we need to exercise for half an hour per session and do that three times per week, we are looking at an hour and a half. Written down, that does not sound that much, but it feels a lot when you do not want to do it.

Even one and a half hours is not the real cost of exercising, though. If I am going running, I need to put my running gear on, stretch up, go for the run, come home, have a shower and wash my running gear. That stacks up: I might spend an hour on completing my 30-minute run task.

Running is one of the best for time ratios. If I am going to the gym, or a team sport activity, there is also travel time and other factors to include. Suddenly this commitment to exercise is stacking up.

This is all fine if we are fired up about exercise. However, a lot of the time we are not. How do we find the motivation go out when we feel this way?

The benefit of habits

If we say we are spending an hour all-inclusive exercising, and we are doing this three times a week, that is a total of three hours per week or just over 25 minutes per day. That sounds like a lot. But how else do we spend our time? Here are my estimates.

Activity	Time per day
Brushing your teeth	6-8 minutes
Showering	15-20 minutes
Cooking and eating	30 minutes-2 hours
Sleeping	7-9 hours

These times are estimates. You may be a quick showerer for example (though you still have to get undressed, dried and dressed again), you may skip breakfast, or you may spend even longer cooking. However, as rough guides, I think they fit.

Put in context, exercise is not *that* time-consuming. Yet, so often, we fail to put in the time. Why? There are two reasons.

One is that some of those tasks we *have* to do. We cannot skip sleeping or eating, for example. Our body will drive us to do these activities if we do not spend enough time on them. They are non-optional. Often, our body even makes them enjoyable. Even showering, which we do not really *need* to do, social convention dictates that we do on a regular basis (and again, a relaxing shower can be enjoyable).

This is not typically true of exercise. Our body does not drive us to exercise. In fact, given the feeling we experience when we start, it feels like it is just the opposite. We can just not do it, and in the short-term, we are fine.

In the long-term, we will not be fine. Therefore a simple solution would be to remind ourselves that exercise *is* non-optional if we want to be healthy. If that works for you, then great, but realistically most of us are not going to be able to talk ourselves into being motivated.

However, there is another important factor at work here. These other activities tend to be habits. No matter what I am doing, my day typically looks like this:

- Get up
- Brush my teeth
- Have some breakfast
- Do some stuff
- Have lunch
- Do some stuff
- Have dinner
- Have a shower
- Brush my teeth
- Go to bed

No matter what else I am doing in my life, I am usually doing these other activities every day. They are habits. I do them on autopilot. I do not think about getting up and brushing my teeth; I just do it while still half-asleep.

The problem with exercise is that most of us do not do it every day. We do it on an ad-hoc basis when we have time, and therefore it is never a habit and always a chore.

Making exercise a habit

If tedious maintenance tasks are easier to do if they are a habit, how can we make exercise a habit?

One option would be to do it every day. This approach is a very simple one as it means you can just get out of bed every morning and do your thing. However, this in itself requires a lot of motivation (every day!) and a lot of time too. Many people just cannot commit to it.

Every week is also useful. Or several times a week. The key here is to have a routine. You want to get to 10 am on Saturday at 7 pm on a Wednesday and think "right, this is when I exercise. If you have a set time, you will think that. If you do not have a set time, you will say "well, I could just go tomorrow instead".

Case study

Every morning Callum would wake up and ask himself "is today a gym day?". More often than not, it turned out that today was not a gym day.

To improve this, and make his life easier, he assigned days: Monday, Wednesday and Friday would now be gym days.

This approach did not magically add any motivation. But it did switch his thoughts from "is today a gym day?" to "ugh, today is a gym day." And even though he may not have been excited about it, he went more often.

What is also important is that he could now wake up on Tuesday, Thursday, Saturday and Sunday and think "today is not a gym day and I do not need to feel guilty about that."

Finding motivation for exercise

Even when you have found the time to exercise, you then actually have to go out and do it. This can be tough, too.

Remind yourself of the memory trap

Earlier we talked about the memory trap. This referred to anxiety being a memory disorder: our minds tell us that an activity will be unrewarding and result in low mood. The reality is that our mood is already low and going out and exercising will improve it.

If you are struggling to get out of the door, remind yourself about the memory trap. Your mind is playing tricks on you. Do not be angry, just smile to yourself, say "thanks, mind" and take a moment to remember that you will feel better once you get out of the door.

One step at a time

My friend Euan is a marathon runner. When he goes out for a run, it really is a run. How does he find the motivation to get himself out the door? He says he doesn't.

He just finds the motivation to put on his running gear. That is all he has to do. Of course, once he has his running gear on, there is nothing else to do but go for a run.

The key for him is that he does not start with the end goal in mind. He does not think about all the pain of running for hours when he is trying to get himself out of the door. He just focuses on the next step: getting his running gear on.

This technique may be useful for you too. Do not spend time dwelling on the whole activity. Focus on the next step. What is the next thing you need to do to accomplish your activity?

There is no pressure to continue after that. If you put your running gear on and then decide not to go for a run that is fine. Of course, you probably will go. In *the causation myth*, we looked at how our thoughts can be driven by our actions. So if we put our running gear on, there will be a good chance our thoughts will follow, and we will go for the run.

The key is that you do not need to find the motivation to do the entire task. Just the next step.

Using a reward system

Remember when we discussed temptation bundling in an earlier chapter? Exercise is an ideal candidate for this. Indeed, it was going to the gym that was studied in the original experiment.

Vary your routine

The human mind has an astounding ability to get bored of anything. When we talk about *dream jobs*, we often say things like "chocolate taster". At the back of our minds, we know that if we did this job, we would get very bored of chocolate very quickly. Even I will admit this, and I spend a significant percentage of my life trying to mainline chocolate into my veins74.

Therefore, when we take something like exercise, that we may not be that motivated to get on with in the first place, how do we sustain our interest when we get bored with it?

One way is to keep your exercising novel. Do different things. The novelty factor will wear off eventually, but if you can keep mixing it up, you can keep it novel. Doing this is tough though: there are only so many machines at the gym. Running is pretty much running.

Another route is to look at what the professionals do. It takes years of training to become a great athlete and typically decades to become world-class. How do professional athletes do it? To an extent, they have a real passion for it, but the mundane repetitions of refining a certain technique will bore anyone eventually.

---

74 I realise that mainline means to inject intravenously, and that being intravenous implies a vein, so I did not need to end the sentence with "into my veins". However, it has more dramatic impact when I add it in anyway.

A better suggestion comes from psychologist Angela Duckworth. She suggests "substitute nuance for novelty"[75]. Take what you are already doing and find a new dimension to it, or find a particular skill within it to refine.

Let's say you are into running. Here are some ways you could mix up your run:

- Change the distance
- Change the route
- Change the surface you run on
- Try interval training

Notice that I am **not** suggesting you try running at different times of the day. This is a common suggestion for "spicing up" exercise. However, it would also mean changing the habit you have set up, and as we have already discussed, this is crucial.

You can change your days and times of course, and it might make sense to do this with seasonal changes: it is more pleasant to run during the day in winter (warmer, lighter) and in the evening during summer (still light, cooler). However, these changes should not be done frequently or without planning. Each time we do, we need to re-establish our habit, which is tough.

Set yourself a goal

Sometimes, exercise can feel very meaningless. Sure, we are improving our overall physical and mental health. And yes, we are improving our mood. These are very immaterial benefits, though. There is no clear goal other than "I will feel better". That is not great motivation.

In such cases, setting yourself a goal can be a useful exercise.

I found this helped with my running. When I wanted to run more regularly, I set myself a goal of running the Abbey Dash, a 10km road race that takes place in Leeds each year. I was only running 5km runs at the time, so this seemed a sensible goal I could work towards.

---

75 Stephen J. Dubner. How to Get More Grit in Your Life. Freakonomics Radio. 4 May 2016.

My plan was to increase my distance 0.5km every two weeks until I had built up to the full distance. As it happened it worked too well: feeling great I went out and ran 7km one week, and the full 10km a few weeks later.

Years later when I found that my running had started to drop off again, I decided it was time to set a new goal. I signed up for the Leeds Half Marathon and over a period of 10 weeks built up from running 10km to 20km.

A half marathon is 21km, but I thought the adrenaline would carry me through. As it happens, on the day of the marathon we had a heatwave in Leeds, and the 8-10 degrees Celsius of my training was replaced by 25 degrees Celsius blazing sun. I did finish but physically could not stand for a good 15 minutes after!

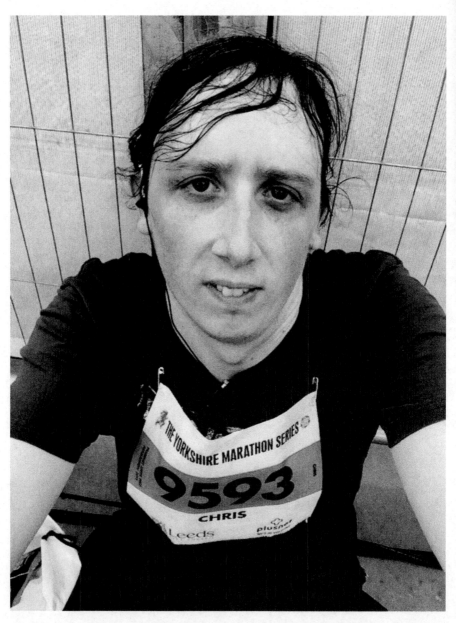

Running is one example, but I have no doubt you will have little trouble dreaming up some goals for whatever exercise you are doing.

Do not forget the original motivation

One point I will caveat this with is that you should not forget why you originally started exercising: to reduce your anxiety and feel better. This may not be a great goal for aiming torwards but it is important not to forget about it.

I came up against this challenge a few years ago when I was thinking about Parkrun. Originally I would drive to the park, do the run and drive back. However, I realised that the park was only 2.5km away, so running there, doing the run and running home would only be a 10km run in total, which was well within my personal range.

There was only one problem, though. The journey to the park may have only been 2.5km away, but it was 2.5km uphill, and the hill got steeper and steeper as you approached the park. This meant I would be exhausted by the time I got to the park and ruin any chance I had of obtaining a new personal best time.

I had a decision to make. Did I want to double my exercise (running 10km instead of 5km) to improve my health, or did I want to achieve my goal of setting a new personal best?

In the end, I decided that although achieving a new personal best would have been nice, the real reason I exercised was to stay healthy. Therefore I decided I would start running to and from Parkrun.

As it turns out, the story has a double happy ending. Not only did I make the correct decision, but it did not hurt my times. The 2.5km did tire me out but also proved an effective warm-up. A few months after I started running to and from Parkrun, I did manage to set a new personal best.

Conquering embarrassment

Many people feel embarrassed about exercising. If you have ever been put off exercising because you are worried that people will make comments or that you will run into someone you know and it will be awkward, you are not alone. Lots of people feel the same way.

Guess what, though? It is your anxiety talking.

People get embarrassed about exercise for a variety of reasons. Some seem to make more sense than others. If you are overweight, you may worry that people will comment on your body shape for example. This is less common than you might think but does sadly happen from time to time.

For others, it is just an unexplainable feeling of dread. You may come up with reasons why it would be embarrassing, but really you just feel like it would be. This feeling is very common but is also textbook anxiety.

What can we do about it? Correctly labelling it as our anxiety talking. That will help us break the anxiety cycle and help us to relax. This approach will only take us so far, though.

Another option is to treat this as a high anxiety situation and look at what we would do for any other scenario: use graded exposure. How can we break the task down and make it more bearable before working up to *full* exposure?

We could start by asking a friend or family member to exercise with us. There is strength in numbers. Or we could find a local running or swimming club and again become part of a group.

Or, if you prefer to do things on your own, you could travel to a park to exercise. Sure, you might want to run around the streets round your house, but if you feel more secure in a park, or that it is more socially acceptable to exercise there, there is no shame in driving there to do your exercise.

Gym visits

Visiting the gym avoids the embarrassment of exercising in public because everyone there is there for the same thing. However, it brings a whole host of other potential worries, especially if you are not a seasoned gym visitor.

Gyms are full of strange equipment. It may be obvious how they work once you know how to use them, but not always before. Maybe you worry you will look silly trying to use them. Or maybe you feel embarrassed that you just wander around without much of a plan while everyone else in there seems to have some professional-grade daily gym routine.

This may be true for a select few, but mostly this is our anxiety talking. All gyms offer an induction, so make sure you take advantage of that. You may also want to plan your gym routine before you go if it helps you feel better about it.

This is not a perfect solution, though, because you may get there and find all the machines are full. Or maybe some of them are out-of-action. The best-laid plans of mice and men often go awry. So be prepared to change your plan if necessary.

Birth plan

When you are expecting a baby, you get two pieces of advice. One is that you should draw up a birth plan. The other is that things almost never go to plan, so do not get too protective over your birth plan.

The whole process felt frustrating to me. What was the point of having a birth plan if we almost certainly could not stick to it?

After much thought, we finally came up with a birth plan we were happy with it. It had three steps in it. "1. Go to the hospital. 2. Have the baby. 3. Come home." The plan worked, and we did not have to stress out that our birth plan was getting derailed.

Where possible, try and keep flexibility in your plan. A lot of anxiety results from us telling ourselves that things have to go according to our plan, things not going to plan, and then us stressing out about it. It is our need to be in control.

Having a flexible plan helps us avoid this headache.

Financial considerations

Many sports you can enjoy for free. However, we should not underestimate our ability to spend money when we do not need to. The UK alone buys two million litres of bottled water every year[76], and that stuff literally falls from the sky and flows out of our taps.

Whatever sport you are doing, there probably someone spending more money than you on it. Running, a sport that should cost you nothing, has an almost endless array of products:

- Running trainers
- Cushioned socks
- Shorts, leggings, tops for all weather
- Running headphones integrated into headbands
- GPS devices and heart monitors
- Wristbands

One of the most striking examples of cycling. The sport is huge in the UK, especially since we began dominating world cycling[77], so cycling clubs are often full of middle-aged men riding £4,000 carbon fibre machines.

------

76 Water Vital Statistics: Industry Data. British Bottled Water Producers. 3 November 2016.

77 Tour de France 2016: How Chris Froome won third yellow jersey. BBC Sport. 24 July 2016. http://www.bbc.co.uk/sport/cycling/36648909

If you are just getting back into cycling, or just taking it up for the first time, the sensible thing to do is to buy a £150 mountain bike on eBay and find out exactly how interested you are in it. But it can be awkward turning up to a cycling club on said bike when everyone else is riding some top-of-the-range bike.

This may or may not be the case. There is nothing to stop you contacting the club in advance to ask what the typical situation is. Often clubs have several ability groups: the A group might be riding 100 miles on carbon fibre beasts, but the C group is probably taking a much more leisurely ride on whatever bikes they happen to own.

Summary of embarrassment

To sum up this section on embarrassment, I want to say that the message here is the same message I push for most of the book: it is entirely normal to feel embarrassed and awkward in these situations. But, the critical thing to remember is, it is your anxiety talking.

Tracking your exercise

You need to monitor how much exercise you do. This needs to be done in a measurable way. For example, tracking it in your head is not going to cut it. Anxiety is a memory disorder. It is too easy to trick yourself into think you have done more.

Therefore, the only way we can get accurate results about how much exercise we are doing is to write it down.

This monitoring can be as simple as keeping a journal. Record what time you start and what time you stop. Use the notes section on your phone, so you can do it while exercising.

An even better way is to use an app on your phone. Both Strava[78] and MapMyFitness[79] are popular. These apps will track your workouts including duration, calories burnt, distance covered, a map of where you went.

---

78 Strava, https://www.strava.com/

79 MapMyFitness, http://www.mapmyfitness.com/

Last Week

 Ran 7.67 km on 07/01/2017 07/01/2...
00:41:48   7.7 km   5:27 min/km

 Ran 5.29 km on 01/01/2017 01/01/2...
00:29:13   5.3 km   5:31 min/km

 Ran 5.25 km on 01/01/2017 01/01/2...
00:29:42   5.3 km   5:39 min/km

Last 30 Days

 Ran 7.45 km on 31/12/2016 31/12/2...
00:41:32   7.4 km   5:34 min/km

 Ran 10.04 km on 25/12/2016 25/12/2...
00:54:19   10.0 km   5:24 min/km

 Ran 5.23 km on 24/12/2016 24/12/2...
00:33:25   5.2 km   6:23 min/km

 Ran 12.00 km on 17/12/2016 17/12/2...
01:03:50   12.0 km   5:19 min/km

 FEED   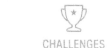 CHALLENGES   +   **WORKOUTS**   ○ ○ ○ MORE

They also give you the ability to share your workouts via Facebook. Doing this is a good way to get support and encouragement from friends.

Exercise in everyday life

Exercise does not just have to take the form of scheduled activities. You can also find ways to be more active in your everyday life. Here are some examples:

- Take the stairs instead of the lift
- Switch your commute or shopping trips to walking
- Do more gardening

Don't mind me; I'm Amish

I always take the stairs instead of using the lift. Most people attribute to wanting to be healthier, but just occasionally somebody will ask for confirmation. "Are you just trying to be healthier?"

Often, I cannot resist a bit of playful teasing. "Oh, my family is Amish" I reply. "We do not believe in using machines that replace the work of man."

Most people would say I am obviously not Amish. I work with computers all day, for example. However, in today's politically correct culture, it is often too embarrassing for people to call you on it, as at the back of their mind they are worried about the fact I might be telling the truth. Accusing someone of lying about their heritage would indeed be a faux pas.

A few do go as far as to question in, though. I get the occasional "really? But you work with computers?" The story has grown more elaborate over time. "Yes" I reply, "but a computer enhances the ability of man, it does not replace it. I could not have a video chat with someone on the other side of the world without a computer. However, I can walk up the stairs without the aid of a lift."

And that is the story of how you can do more exercise in everyday life, while convincing half of the people in your office that you are Amish...

Traps to watch out for

As anxiety sufferers, it is easy to get tricked by our mind. It can take something we are doing for something for a positive reason and turn it around to something negative. Here are some traps to avoid.

Monitoring your weight

The first thing that people do when they start exercising more is jumping on the scales every day. There are a number of problems with doing this.

Exercise does not necessarily help with weight loss[80]. Exercising, especially sports like running and cycling use a lot of energy, but your body makes up for it by eating more. Therefore exercise is only an effective weight loss measure when combined with a programme of diet.

It is often said that muscle weighs more than fat. The reality is more complicated than that[81], but it is true that if you are already quite slim and start exercising more, your weight may go up.

But regardless of what happens to your weight, the danger is that if you start measuring it, it can become a source of anxiety in itself. As if we do not have enough worries already, it is easy to find ourselves getting on the scales every day in an unhealthy obsession with numbers.

You might think "sure, but at least I will lose weight", but this picture is not clear either. Recording your weight is a feature of most diets. However, the evidence that daily weighings helps you lose weight is limited[82].

Your weight fluctuates over the course of a day, and over the course of a week, too[83]. Therefore, weighing yourself more than once per week, on different days, or at different times, may give you misleading results.

When we factor in our predisposition to worry, this seems like a dangerous path to go down. Remember that we are exercising to manage our mental health, rather than just to lose weight.

Learning the hard way

---

80 Denis Campbell. Exercise is good ... but it won't help you lose weight, say doctors. The Guardian. 22 April 2015.

81 William Sukala. Does Muscle Weigh More Than Fat? Weight Watchers. https://www.weightwatchers.com/util/art/index_art.aspx?tabnum=1&art_id=8311&sc=128

82 NHS Choices. Behind the Headlines: Weighing yourself every day may help with weight loss. 19 June 2015. http://www.nhs.uk/news/2015/06June/Pages/Weighing-yourself-everyday-helps-with-weight-loss.aspx

83 Luisa Dillner. How often should I weigh myself? The Guardian. 11 January 2015.

It took me a while to take my own advice on this one. At the start of 2016, I got on the scales for the first time in a long time and found that I was 9kg heavier than when I last weighed myself. This change took my BMI from the nice green zone into the overweight category.

As someone who cooks at home a lot and exercises regularly, this was a depressing sight. It did not seem fair that I was doing all of these good behaviours and was still heavier than I should be.

I then spent the next three months worrying about my weight and counting my calories. It was successful in the short term, dropping me down 8kg84. However, I then went on my honeymoon and put 2kg back on in a week.

A much better idea would have simply been not to look. It was clear by looking at me that I was not significantly overweight. Stress is not healthy, either.

Spending money

I often say that being that running a gym must be one of the most profitable things you can do. They are expensive. The fancy gyms charge people £80 a month or more. For the privilege of paying that, patrons often have to sign up for a 12-month contract.

How do people react to this? Do they become angry, demand lower prices and shorter contracts? No. They say "oh, paying that much and forcing me to pay it for an entire year will definitely motivate me to go on a regular basis."

Then they sign up, go for a few weeks, get fed up with it and rarely go again. The gym owner continues to collect their £1,000 in total yearly fees from someone who rarely ever visits your facilities.

It is weird because human psychology rarely works this way. It is called "sunk cost fallacy". People generally try and get their money's worth whatever the cost. But visiting the gym is the one area of life where people seem to avoid this trap.

What is sunk cost fallacy?

---

84 Chris Worfolk. Slimming down. 14 July 2016.
http://blog.chrisworfolk.com/2016/07/14/slimming-down/

Sunk cost fallacy is all about try to get value for money that you have already lost. For example, let's say you go to the cinema. You spend £10 on your ticket and then half way through realise that the film is boring and that you are not enjoying it.

Do you walk out? Most people say no. They want to get their money's worth. But this does not make any sense. The money is gone. You cannot get your £10 back. The only choice you have is whether to waste the next hour of your life or not. Most of us just sit there to "get our money's worth".

A study in America looked at exactly this issue85. They tracked people on a $70 gym subscription to see how often they visited. On average, they went so rarely that switching to the $10 pay-per-visit option would save them $17 per gym trip.

Spending money does not provide motivation to exercise. Or anything else for that matter. The reason is that when you get *the prize* at the start, you get a little dopamine release. This makes you feel like you have achieved something and reduces your motivation to finish it86.

When I was learning to play the guitar, I could have just gone out and bought myself a new Fender Telecaster. I had seen the research, though, and was keen the avoid this trap. Instead, I told myself that if I practised for an hour per day, for 60 days, I would be allowed to buy myself the new guitar.

Was my old guitar harder to play? It really was. Did the exercise work, though? You bet it did. In fact, I managed to practice for two hours per day and the feeling of buying my Telecaster at the end of it was amazing87.

85 Stefano DellaVigna, Ulrike Malmendier. Paying Not to Go to the Gym. JEL D00, D12, D91.

86 Derek Sivers. Keep your goals to yourself. TEDGlobal 2010.

87 Chris Worfolk, "Fender Telecaster", http://blog.chrisworfolk.com/2014/03/09/fender-telecaster/

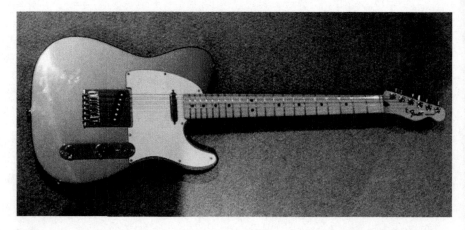

What should we take from this research? That the gym membership, the ultimate reward, should come **after** you have started your exercise routine, and not before. Set yourself a goal, such as a new fitness routine, and use the reward of a gym membership as the motivation to stick to it.

Mindfulness in exercise

As we know, mindfulness is about living in the moment and enjoying our everyday experiences. For some exercise, we get this out-of-the-box. In team sports for example, your head is likely to be so far in the game that you do not have time for other thoughts.

With solo exercises, such as walking, running, cycling and swimming, it is easier for our mind to drift off and unpleasant thoughts to intrude.

Mindfulness teaches us that we need to allow these thoughts to come and go. We should not resist them, but we should not hold onto them, either.

If you are out walking or running, this is an excellent chance to practice mindfulness. Take the time to look around you. Breath in the air; take in the sights. What can you hear? What can you smell? What can you see?

If you usually exercise with your headphones in, consider leaving them at home. Or, practice mindfulness for the first half of your exercise routine, and then put your headphones in for the other half.

Summary

In this chapter, we learnt that exercise is one of the most effective ways of treating anxiety. We looked at how much exercise we need to do and how intense it has to be.

Importantly, we learnt that to exercise on a regular basis, we need to make it a habit. We need an exercise *routine*. It needs to be something that is easy to stick to it. It is better to start slow and build up.

Action steps

- Track your exercise using a journal or phone app.
- Ensure the amount of time you spend exercising is at least the minimum recommended. Do this by looking at the actual numbers that you are tracking and not your memory.

If you decide to do more exercise:

- Select something that you will enjoy doing, to keep you motivated.
- Ask yourself "how can I make this a habit or routine?"
- Set yourself a goal, if appropriate.

Start off slow and build up. That means going to the gym once a week at first, then twice a week once you have proven you can consistently do it once per week. It also means spending as little as possible until you have proven to yourself that you can stick with it.

Diet

Food, glorious food. Who does not enjoy a hot sausage with mustard?

Diet is obviously a significant factor in your physical health. Along with exercise, it was one the two things people think about when trying to lead a healthier life: "eat right and exercise more".

What you might not realise is just how important diet is mental health as well. Here is how a paper in *The Lancet* described the importance of diet88.

"Evidence is steadily growing for the relation between dietary quality (and potential nutritional deficiencies) and mental health, and for the select use of nutrient-based supplements to address deficiencies, or as monotherapies or augmentation therapies. We advocate recognition of diet and nutrition as central determinants of both physical and mental health."

Studies consistently find a relationship between poor diet and poor mental health89. Therefore, a healthy diet is a cornerstone of managing anxiety through lifestyle.

Why is a healthy diet good for mental health?

Studies agree that a healthy balanced diet correlated with good mental health. The exact reasons for this are not entirely clear90. However, the link is strong enough for us to say that it is clear that a proper diet is a contributing factor to making us feel well91.

Eating well also comes with some other related benefits:

---

88 Sarris, Jerome et al. Nutritional medicine as mainstream in psychiatry. The Lancet Psychiatry, Volume 2, Issue 3, 271-274

89 O'Neil A, Quirk SE, Housden S, et al. Relationship Between Diet and Mental Health in Children and Adolescents: A Systematic Review. American Journal of Public Health. 2014;104(10):e31-e42. doi:10.2105/AJPH.2014.302110.

90 Kenneth R Fox. The influence of physical activity on mental well-being. Public Health Nutrition, Volume 2, Issue 3a. March 1999, pp. 411-418. DOI: https://doi.org/10.1017/S1368980099000567

91 Dr Ursula Werneke. Eating well and mental health. Royal College of Psychiatrists. January 2014.

- A healthy diet improves our physical health92, which makes us feel better and improves our mood.
- A healthy diet makes it less likely we will become ill93.
- A healthy diet improves your mood94.

What should I eat?

There are no specific "mental health" foods. In this respect, when I talk about a healthy balanced diet, I am talking about the same thing everyone else is talking about. A healthy diet for us is the same as a healthy diet for a muggle.

Let's briefly remind ourselves of the basics of healthy eating:

- Fruit and vegetables are good. Do not get too hung up on the idea of having five portions of fruit and veg per day. Five is just a marketing number. The reality is that more is good, less is bad. If you have four portions per day you have not "failed"; it is better than having none. However, if you have eight portions, that is better than five.
- Plenty of carbohydrates like whole grains and rice are good95.
- Fat and sugar should be eaten in moderation96.
- Red meat should be eaten in moderation97.

---

92 Harvard Medical School. Making Sense of Vitamins and Minerals: Choosing the foods and nutrients you need to stay healthy

93 Mente A, de Koning L, Shannon HS, Anand SS. A Systematic Review of the Evidence Supporting a Causal Link Between Dietary Factors and Coronary Heart Disease. Arch Intern Med. 2009;169(7):659-669. doi:10.1001/archinternmed.2009.38

94 Annette Dunne. Food and mood: evidence for diet-related changes in mental health. British Journal of Community Nursing. Nov 2012 Nutrition Supplement, pS20-S24. DOI: http://dx.doi.org/10.12968/bjcn.2012.17.Sup11.S20

95 NHS Choices, "Eating a balanced diet", http://www.nhs.uk/Livewell/Goodfood/Pages/Healthyeating.aspx

96 Dr Alison Tedstone, Victoria Targett, Dr Rachel Allen. Sugar Reduction: The evidence for action. Public Health England. October 2015.

97 Sabine Rohrmann, Kim Overvad, H Bas Bueno-de-Mesquita, Marianne U Jakobsen, Rikke Egeberg, Anne Tjønneland, Laura Nailler, Marie-Christine Boutron-Ruault, Françoise Clavel-Chapelon, Vittorio Krogh, Domenico Palli, Salvatore Panico, Rosario Tumino, Fulvio Ricceri, Manuela M Bergmann, Heiner Boeing, Kuanrong Li, Rudolf Kaaks, Kay-Tee Khaw, Nicholas J Wareham, Francesca L Crowe, Timothy J Key, Androniki Naska, Antonia Trichopoulou, Dimitirios Trichopoulos, Max Leenders, Petra

- Processed meat should be eaten only infrequently98.
- Fast food should be eaten only infrequently99.

Getting your five-a-day

My friends Katie and Joe turned their quest to eat plenty of fruit and vegetables into a competition. Each day they would attempt to out-do each other in how many portions they could eat. They purchased all kind of weird and wonderful vegetables to get ahead of each other.

It was all in good fun of course, and they both ended up eating a lot easier because of it. Could you challenge someone you know to a similar competition?

Rules of thumb

There are specific amounts of each type of food that seem to be optimal for your body. However, can you imagine sitting down to work this out every day? Making sure you get exactly the right amount of vitamin A, the exact right amount of protein and the exact right amount of fat?

That would be time-consuming for muggles, but for those of us with anxiety, it could quickly become an obsession and constant source of worry.

Therefore, to avoid getting too hung up on this, let's just avoid the subject altogether. Instead, let's have some *rules of thumb* by which to try and plan our diet. Here are mine:

HM Peeters, Dagrun Engeset, Christine L Parr, Guri Skeie, Paula Jakszyn, María-José Sánchez, José M Huerta, M Luisa Redondo, Aurelio Barricarte, Pilar Amiano, Isabel Drake, Emily Sonestedt, Göran Hallmans, Ingegerd Johansson, Veronika Fedirko, Isabelle Romieux, Pietro Ferrari, Teresa Norat, Anne C Vergnaud, Elio Riboli and Jakob Linseisen. Meat consumption and mortality - results from the European Prospective Investigation into Cancer and Nutrition. BMC Medicine 2013 11:63. DOI: 10.1186/1741-7015-11-63

98 Véronique Bouvard, Dana Loomis, Kathryn Z Guyton, Yann Grosse, Fatiha El Ghissassi, Lamia Benbrahim-Tallaa, Neela Guha, Heidi Mattock, Kurt Straif. Carcinogenicity of consumption of red and processed meat. The Lancet Oncology. Volume 16, No. 16, p1599–1600, December 2015. DOI: http://dx.doi.org/10.1016/S1470-2045(15)00444-1

99 Panel on Dietetic Products, Nutrition and Allergies. Scientific Opinion on Dietary Reference Values for fats, including saturated fatty acids, polyunsaturated fatty acids, monounsaturated fatty acids, trans fatty acids, and cholesterol. European Food Safety Authority. EFSA Journal 2010; 8(3):1461 107 pp. DOI: 10.2903/j.efsa.2010.1461

1.   Vegetables or salad with every meal
2.   Red meat a maximum of twice a week
3.   At least one vegetarian meal a week

I do not always hit them, and I do not stress about it too much when I miss. But they form a useful guide to whether I am in the correct area or not.

Measuring your diet

As I discussed above, there are two metrics we want to factor in when we measure our diet:

- Am I eating a sensible amount of food (how many kcals)?
- Am I eating a suitable balance of different foods?

As explained in the previous section, having some rules of thumb of measuring these is the best way forward. We do not want this to become a source of anxiety in itself.

For example, you can often measure whether you are eating a good balance of different food groups simply by counting the number of different colours on your plate. The more you have, the better you are doing, generally speaking.

However, if you want to go deeper into it, there are tools to help you do this. Probably the easiest way is to download an app to your mobile phone that allows you to input what you are eating, and it will track the food groups and calories for you.

Two popular apps are:

- myfitnesspal100
- LifeSum101

Entering what you eat into these apps will give you an approximate calorie count and breakdown of the types of food you are eating. Beware, though: these figures may not be accurate unless you can find an exact product/brand match. Do not forget to include any snacks you have, and any drinks other than water.

---

100 myfitnesspal, https://www.myfitnesspal.com/

101 LifeSum, https://lifesum.com/

I find measuring my diet is useful for a short period. I might do it for a week or two to get a picture, but then stop myself from recording any further to prevent it from becoming an obsession.

However, there are specific things you may want to measure if you are looking to improve them. For example:

- How often you have eaten junk food
- How often you snack on chocolate or sugar
- How often you eat red meat
- How often you drink alcohol

Remember that anxiety is a memory disorder. It is easy to downplay the bad habits that plague our lives. Our memory will tell us it is not as bad as we think it is. But written-down numbers do not lie. They provide us with an accurate measure of how well we are doing.

How much should I eat?

Food intake is usually measured in kilocalories, known as kcals for short. The headline for our suggested intake of these are as follows:

Gender	Daily kcals
Men	2,500
Women	2,000

These numbers are misleading, though, because the amount you need to consume is affected by your lifestyle as well as your gender. For example, I work in an office and do little manual labour, so an intake of 1,800 may be sufficient for me to maintain my weight.

Quick wins

There are some easy ways to improve your diet in a short amount of time. Perhaps the best is swapping certain foods out for more nutritious alternatives. Here are some ways you can do this:

Item	Swap it for
White bread	Brown bread
White rice	Brown rice
Sugary cereal	Plain cereal
Cans of pop	Sugar-free versions
Juice	No added sugar juice

Crisps	Unsalted nuts
Whole milk	Skimmed milk
Baked potato with cheese	Baked potato with avocado
Chips	Boiled potatoes

Best of all, here is my top tip from *Technical Anxiety* 102.

"If you go out for dinner or drinks, swap your coke for half coke, half diet coke. If they look at you strangely, explain that you are trying to watch your figure."

If you are not familiar with the reference, it is from a Tenacious D song 103. But also an excellent way to reduce your calories.

Out-of-date food

I have a strained relationship with best-before and use-by dates. Supermarkets print these on products to give you a guide to when food starts to go bad. However, it is in their interest to be over-cautious to avoid lawsuits and to sell more food 104.

So, what are you supposed to be with a packet of vegetables or piece of chicken that was supposed to be eaten by yesterday?

For a muggle, this would be a simple decision: you either decide it eat it or throw it away. However, when you add anxiety into the mix, you then have to consider whether you are throwing it away because you genuinely should, or because you are letting your anxiety win.

Perhaps the question of whether throwing away chicken is proof that anxiety is controlling your life is over thinking the situation. But over thinking the situation is what anxiety is all about.

102 Chris Worfolk. Technical Anxiety: The complete guide to what is anxiety and what to do about it. ISBN: 978-1539424215

103 Tenacious D. Drive-Thru. Tenacious D (album). Epic Records. 25 September 2001.

104 Joanna Blythman. Why supermarkets' love of use-by dates leads to food waste. The Guardian. 4 November 2015.

Throwing the food away is a sensible option. Food is cheaper now than it has ever been105. Therefore, assuming you are not eating wagyu steak or fresh truffle, it is hardly a big waste of money to throw out-of-date food away. You may decide that a little more money and a lot less worry is worth it.

Another option is to use this as an opportunity to challenge your anxiety. Give the item a good eyeball, and a good sniff, and if it passes both tests, eat it. This behaviour is exposure. We are training our brain that we can eat without coming down with food poisoning.

A final option is to feed the potentially-bad food to your dog, partner, child, etc. This way you can see it is safe before consuming it yourself. Bare in mind though that if they do die, "yeah, I knew the food was poisoned" is a weak defence when brought before a jury.

As a caveat, I will add that the official recommendation from the NHS is not to eat any food past its "use-by" date106. Do not get this confused with other terms, though. You can safely ignore these:

- "Best before"
- "Display until"
- "Sell by"

Planning for a healthy diet

A healthy diet rarely happens by accident. In fact, the opposite is true: unhealthy eating is typically a result of us not planning or thinking about our diet.

Developing a meal plan

The majority of unhealthy dinners that I have are a result of lack of planning. It is the days when I realise I do not have a recipe ready, so to make things easier I pull the chips out of the freezer, order takeaway, or drive to the nearest fried chicken outlet.

---

105 Rob Lyons. Panic on a Plate: How Society Developed an Eating Disorder. 1 October 2011. ISBN: 1845402162

106 NHS Choices, "Food labelling terms", http://www.nhs.uk/Livewell/Goodfood/Pages/food-labelling-terms.aspx

To avoid myself falling into this trap, I sit down once a week and write out a meal plan. This details lunch and dinner for each day. I then order the ingredients I need for everything from the supermarket and schedule a delivery.

Day	Lunch	Dinner
Saturday		
Sunday		
Monday		
Tuesday		
Wednesday		
Thursday		
Friday		

Each day, I look at the meal plan, which tells me what I am making and where I can find the recipe, then it is simply a case of following the plan.

This approach is similar to the habits we talked about in the chapter on exercise. If I just decided what to cook on a night I would say things like:

- "I cannot be bothered to make anything complicated tonight"
- "I do not have the ingredients I need for that"
- "I am busy; it will be easier to order in takeaway"

However, if I already have a plan in place, I do not have to subject myself to the cognitive load of making this decision. I just follow the plan out of a habit and end up with a better diet because of it.

Other dietary factors

Diet is not just about food. It also covers the other things we put in our body: such as water, alcohol and other substances. These too play a part in affecting our mental health.

Hydration

What if there was a magic cure for anxiety where all you had to do was drink a glass of water every day, and you would feel better. Well, there is, and it is exactly that. It has to be a gigantic glass if that is all you are drinking per day, but an easier approach is to re-fill a smaller glass several times.

Drinking water itself is not going to be a magic cure for your anxiety. However, it has been shown that not staying hydrated leads to poor mental health[107], as well as poor physical health.

How much should you drink? There is no specific guidance, but typically around 6-8 glasses of water per day is a good amount[108]. Who has time to measure that, though? Your urine will be your best clue. The lighter it is, the more hydrated you are. A darker coloured urine suggests you are not drinking enough.

There is no upper limit. You cannot drink too much water. Your body can to regulate its amount of water, so it is not something you can overdose on. So just keep drinking.

Drugs and water regulation

There is one exception to the "no such thing as too much water" rule. Certain drugs, such as ecstasy, interfere with the body's ability to regulate its water levels[109]. Therefore, if you are consuming such a substance, you need to be a little more careful.

If you do not like the taste of water (I do not), you want to make sure you can get your liquid without also doing damage. For example, you could drink nothing but Coca-Cola, or coffee, and get the water you need, but also a lorry-load of sugar and caffeine too. No added sugar fruit juice and fruit tea are much better options.

---

107 Josef Brown, Glenn Marland. Hydration in older people with mental health problems. Nursing Times, Volume 3, Page 38.

108 NHS Choices, "Water, drinks and your health", http://www.nhs.uk/Livewell/Goodfood/Pages/water-drinks.aspx

109 The Association of the British Pharmaceutical Industry, "ADH and control of the water balance", http://www.abpischools.org.uk/page/modules/homeostasis_kidneys/kidneys6.cfm

Barriers to hydration

It is easy not to drink enough water. However, for most of us, it is not that do not want to drink water, or do not feel thirsty: it is just that we forget.

Or, that we are sat at our desks, or out and about, and do not want to interrupt our activity to go drink something. Life rarely comes with scheduled water breaks (unlike when you play team sports, for example, in which a good coach will explicitly include these).

We can solve both of these problems by keeping water to hand. Carry a bottle of water around with you. You do not need **bottled** water. Just get a water bottle and re-fill it from your tap. Carry it around and make sure there are no barriers to you staying hydrated.

Alcohol

"To alcohol! The cause of... and solution to... all of life's problems." Homer Simpson.

Two situations are very common for people with anxiety: people who have a drinking problem[110] and people who drink no alcohol. Sometimes it is both.

It is easy to see how both arrive. Anxiety is a depressant: it relaxes you. Therefore, even if you have never heard of anxiety before and have no idea you have it, it is pretty easy to make the connection between consuming a large amount of alcohol and feeling better.

The scary part is: it works. Alcohol is often an incredibly efficient way to self-medicate, so many people do it[111]. The problem, like any medication, is that it comes with a lot of side-effects. In the case of alcohol, these can be particularly destructive.

I am certainly not advocating using alcohol to manage your anxiety. However, if you do engage in such behaviours, I think it is important that you know that:

---

110 Grant BF, Stinson FS, Dawson DA, et al. Prevalence and Co-occurrence of Substance Use Disorders and IndependentMood and Anxiety Disorders: Results From the National Epidemiologic Survey on Alcohol and RelatedConditions. Arch Gen Psychiatry. 2004;61(8):807-816. doi:10.1001/archpsyc.61.8.807.

111 Kushner MG, Sher KJ, Beitman BD. The relation between alcohol problems and the anxiety disorders. Am J Psychiatry. 1990 Jun;147(6):685-95. DOI: 10.1176/ajp.147.6.685

- You are not alone.
- Your drinking and your anxiety may well be related.

If you do find you are struggling with alcohol, the first step would usually be to talk your GP about it. They can help you tackle your drinking and your anxiety. If you feel uncomfortable about this, there are independent charities who specialise in alcohol abuse.

Other people may find they have the opposite problem. They have stopped drinking because they were advised by their doctor, or because they do not like feeling out-of-control. This makes sense because our anxiety is often about wanting to be in control. Many anxiety sufferers do not drink, even though they would like to, and feel like they are letting their anxiety win by **not** drinking.

Perhaps the real question is, should we be drinking, and if so, how much?

From a health point of view, the evidence is mixed. You would expect the answer to be clear. After all, alcohol is a poison. That is probably the reason it tastes so horrible when you first start drinking. You have to train your taste buds to accept it. Therefore, it should be bad for you.

But it isn't. Time and time again studies show that people who are moderate drinkers live the longest[112]. Heavy drinkers die younger than moderate drinkers do. But nobody, even the heavy drinkers, die as young as the non-drinkers.

Successive studies keep controlling for more and more factors, such as pre-existing health conditions, but the evidence keeps pointing to alcohol being good for you.

Why? The truth is, we do not know. These are cohort studies, so cannot point to direct cause and effect. The most convincing argument I have heard so far is that people who drink will often do so socially, and the benefit of going out and having friends[113], especially in later life[114], is massive.

---

112 Holahan, C. J., Schutte, K. K., Brennan, P. L., Holahan, C. K., Moos, B. S. and Moos, R. H. (2010), Late-Life Alcohol Consumption and 20-Year Mortality. Alcoholism: Clinical and Experimental Research, 34: 1961–1971. doi:10.1111/j.1530-0277.2010.01286.x

113 Sayette MA, Creswell KG, Dimoff JD, Fairbairn CE, Cohn JF, Heckman BW, Kirchner TR, Levine JM, Moreland RL. Alcohol and group formation: a multimodal investigation of

Whatever the cause, the evidence can be denied no longer. Muggles should drink alcohol. It is good for them.

For anxiety sufferers, there is an extra layer to consider. Alcohol can increase your anxiety, and as this has a measurable effect on our quality of life, this needs to be factored into the calculation.

Here again, though, the evidence suggests we might be better off drinking. A 2009 study suggested that moderate alcohol consumption was better than low alcohol consumption for both anxiety and depression[115].

Therefore, the evidence suggests that if you can drink in moderation, you should. Or at least, there is no evidence that you **should not** drink unless you fall into the problem-drinking category.

How much alcohol should I drink?

The research is clear that the best results from alcohol are achieving by consuming it in moderation. So how much is too much? There are no specific guidelines for alcohol regarding anxiety, so we have to use the recommended guidelines for a typical person.

These vary from country to country. Here are the current guidelines for the UK[116] which are a good benchmark:

- No more than 14 units per week
- Consumption should be spread out across several days
- There should be some "alcohol-free" days

Units can be a confusing term, so here are the number of units per week translated into real terms:

---

the effects of alcohol on emotion and social bonding. Psychol Sci. 2012 Aug 1;23(8):869-78. doi: 10.1177/0956797611435134.

114 Andrew Steptoe, Aparna Shankar, Panayotes Demakakos, and Jane Wardle. Social isolation, loneliness, and all-cause mortality in older men and women. PNAS vol. 110 no. 15. DOI: 10.1073/pnas.1219686110

115 Skogen JC, Harvey SB, Henderson M, Stordal E, Mykletun A. Anxiety and depression among abstainers and low-level alcohol consumers. The Nord-Trøndelag Health Study. Addiction. 2009 Sep;104(9):1519-29. doi: 10.1111/j.1360-0443.2009.02659.x.

116 NHS Choices, "Alcohol units", http://www.nhs.uk/Livewell/alcohol/Pages/alcohol-units.aspx

Drink	Units per drink	Weekly recommendation
Beer (3.6%)	2 units	7 pints
Can of larger	2 units	7 cans
Glass of wine	1.5 units	9 glasses
Large glass of wine	2 units	7 glasses
Spirit and mixer	1 unit	14 drinks

Smoking

Smoking is really bad for you[117]. There is no question about whether it takes years off your life, the question is merely whether the effect is five years or ten[118].

I will not spend too much time on this topic because I do not think anyone will find such claims controversial, or dispute the idea that smoking is bad for you.

However, it is worth noting that smoking and anxiety can often be found together. This makes sense because, in the short-term, smoking can relieve anxiety[119]. Therefore, some people may use smoking to self-medicate.

In the long term, smoking seems to be unhelpful for anxiety. In a study looking at the correlation, smokers were found to have higher levels of anxiety than non-smokers[120]. Stopping smoking helped, but did not reduce anxiety to the level of non-smokers.

117 Bjartveit K, Tverdal A. Health consequences of smoking 1–4 cigarettes per day. Tobacco Control. 2005;14(5):315-320. doi:10.1136/tc.2005.011932.

118 Michael Darden, Donna B. Gilleskie, and Koleman Strumpf. Smoking and Mortality: New Evidence from a Long Panel. Department of Economics, Tulane University. January 2016.

119 Damee Choia, Shotaro Otab, Shigeki Watanukia. Does cigarette smoking relieve stress? Evidence from the event-related potential (ERP). International Journal of Psychophysiology. Volume 98, Issue 3, Part 1, December 2015, Pages 470–476. DOI: http://dx.doi.org/10.1016/j.ijpsycho.2015.10.005

120 Mykletun A, Overland S, Aarø LE, Liabø HM, Stewart R. Smoking in relation to anxiety and depression: evidence from a large population survey: the HUNT study. Eur Psychiatry. 2008 Mar;23(2):77-84. Epub 2007 Dec 21. DOI: 10.1016/j.eurpsy.2007.10.005

Illicit drugs

Many people with anxiety will misuse drugs[121]. This is thought to be for the same reason that so many people abuse alcohol: it is a form of self-medication, providing relief from anxiety in the short term.

Given that anxiety can be the cause of drug misuse[122], and that drug misuse can be the cause of anxiety, if you want to tackle them, it is best to tackle both issues together.

A great place to start is by talking to your GP. However, if you feel uncomfortable doing this, most countries have a range of independent charities and organisations that are willing to help.

If you do not have issues with drug misuse and can maintain a *healthy* relationship with them, it is worth us remembering that different drugs carry varying levels of risk.

In 2007, a group of scientists, led by Professor David Nutt (who was famously sacked from his position as a government advisor for pointing out their policies were nonsense[123]), produced an index of how dangerous the most popular drugs were[124]. This is how they ranked:

1. Heroin
2. Cocaine
3. Barbiturates
4. Street methadone
5. Alcohol

---

121 Smith JP, Book SW. Anxiety and Substance Use Disorders: A Review. The Psychiatric times. 2008;25(10):19-23.

122 Grant BF, Stinson FS, Dawson DA, Chou SP, Dufour MC, Compton W, Pickering RP, Kaplan K. Prevalence and co-occurrence of substance use disorders and independent mood and anxiety disorders: results from the National Epidemiologic Survey on Alcohol and Related Conditions. Arch Gen Psychiatry. 2004 Aug;61(8):807-16. DOI: 10.1001/archpsyc.61.8.807

123 Alan Travis. Chief drug adviser David Nutt sacked over cannabis stance. The Guardian. 30 October 2009.

124 Prof David Nutt, Leslie A King, William Saulsbury, Prof Colin Blakemore. Development of a rational scale to assess the harm of drugs of potential misuse. The Lancet. Volume 369, No. 9566, p1047–1053, 24 March 2007. DOI: http://dx.doi.org/10.1016/S0140-6736(07)60464-4

6. Ketamine
7. Benzodiazepines
8. Amphetamines
9. Tobacco
10. Buprenorphine
11. Cannabis
12. Solvents
13. 4-MTA
14. LSD
15. Methylphenidate
16. Anabolic steroids
17. GHB
18. Ecstasy
19. Alkyl Nitrates
20. Khat

There are no surprises at the top of the list. Both heroin125 and cocaine126 are dangerous substances and can kill you. Cannabis may be more of a surprise: it ranks higher than a lot of people expect it to.

Certainly, in the context of anxiety, cannabis is a substance to be avoided. Cannabis use has been shown to correlate with mental health problems127. You could argue that a cohort study does not prove causation. However, the cannabis use was predictive of mental health problems *later* in life, and therefore it is unlikely the cannabis usage was caused by self-medicating existing mental health difficulties.

Other substances, such as LCD and ecstasy come far further down the list. The evidence suggests it is safer to use these drugs than it is to use alcohol

125 Shane Darke and Wayne Hall. Heroin overdose: Research and evidence-based intervention. J Urban Health. 2003 Jun; 80(2): 189–200. DOI: 10.1093/jurban/jtg022

126 Daniel Robaei, Stuart M. Grieve, G.C. Nelson, Ravinay Bhindi, Gemma A. Figtree. Cocaine-induced epicardial coronary artery thrombosis resulting in extensive myocardial injury assessed by cardiac magnetic resonance imaging. European Heart Journal. DOI: http://dx.doi.org/10.1093/eurheartj/ehq229

127 George C Patton, Carolyn Coffey, John B Carlin, Louisa Degenhardt, Michael Lynskey, Wayne Hall. Cannabis use and mental health in young people: cohort study. BMJ 2002;325:1195.

and tobacco. In the case of LCD, there seem to be no long-term health effects128.

Restaurants

Restaurants prove a challenge for us anxiety sufferers in a number of ways. Some of us may worry about the nutritional content of the food. Others may worry about the standards of hygiene in the kitchen. Many of us worry about the experience itself, given that restaurants are almost always social situations.

Are restaurants bad for diet?

The nutritional content of restaurants is not entirely clear. There are a number of potential problems with restaurant food:

- Portion sizes are often unhealthily large.
- They may not contain any vegetables unless specifically ordered.
- Chefs often use cooking techniques that make food less healthy, such as cooking in butter or using lots of salt.

However, for a long time, it was believed that you could eat at restaurants and not gain weight because you compensated by eating less at home.

A 2007 study indicated that eating at restaurants was not associated with weight gain129. However, more recent research published in the journal *Public Health Nutrition* concluded that restaurants were associated with weight gain as people did not compensate130.

---

128 Understanding the mental health effects of street drugs. Mind. 2011. https://www.mind.org.uk/media/158223/understanding_the_mental_health_effect_of_street_drugs_2011.pdf

129 Duffey KJ, Gordon-Larsen P, Jacobs DR Jr, Williams OD, Popkin BM. Differential associations of fast food and restaurant food consumption with 3-y change in body mass index: the Coronary Artery Risk Development in Young Adults Study. Am J Clin Nutr. 2007 Jan;85(1):201-8.

130 Rebecca Smith. Eating in restaurants no better than fast food for health. The Telegraph. 8 August 2016.

One fact that was clear from all of the research was that eating fast food was bad for you, and strongly correlated with weight gain131.

How do restaurant critics stay thin?

When I am not writing books about anxiety, I am writing books about restaurants at home132 and abroad133. When we are working, we eat out a lot. At one point, I was eating out as much as ten times per week. I managed to do this without putting on any significant weight.

How did I do this? I am not sure. Perhaps my worrying burns a lot of calories.

I am not the only one, though. Emily O'Mara ate at every cheeseburger-serving restaurant in Louisville in her quest to find the perfect one134. She put her lack of weight gain down to having "disciplined the fun".

Of course, both of these stories are a sample size of one and may not apply to anyone else. Your experience may be vastly different.

Dieting

This section contains information on diet programmes to lose weight, but also covers a more general topic of making specific changes to your diet. Mostly, I will be telling you why this is a bad idea. It is easy for us anxiety sufferers to get paranoid about certain foods, and most of the time there is no evidence for this.

Speak to your dietician

If you go to your doctor and ask about diet, they may be able to refer you to a dietician. These are good people to speak to. Dietician is a protected term

---

131 Rosenheck R. Fast food consumption and increased caloric intake: a systematic review of a trajectory towards weight gain and obesity risk. Obes Rev. 2008 Nov;9(6):535-47. doi: 10.1111/j.1467-789X.2008.00477.x. Epub 2008 Mar 14. DOI: 10.1111/j.1467-789X.2008.00477.x

132 Chris Worfolk. Leeds Restaurant Guide. 18 August 2013. ISBN: 1500529966

133 Chris Worfolk. Finland Restaurant Guide. 1 September 2015.

134 Stephen J. Dubner. The Cheeseburger Diet. Freakonomics Radio. 10 December 2015.

in the UK135. Here is what the professional body, the British Dietetic Association (BDA) have to say about it:

"Dieticians are the only nutrition professionals to be regulated by law, and are governed by an ethical code to ensure that they always work to the highest standard."

So if anyone tells you they are a nutritionist or nutritional therapist, that is fine, but be clear that they have just made up a name, which has no value, and they may or may not have any qualifications.

Fads and "superfoods"

If someone came up to you and said they could make you rich very quickly for very little effort, you would probably be suspicious. Similarly, when someone tells you that you can cure cancer and live to 100 by eating goji berries, you want to be suspicious as well.

That is not to say that some foods are not better than others. Kale genuinely is very good for you136. But to bang on the same drum I will regularly hit during this chapter, the best diet is one that is varied.

Organic food

The evidence shows that organic food is no better for you137, is no safer, and does not taste any better138. When put to the test, people cannot tell the difference. However, you may think it tastes better because you have paid more for it139.

---

135 The British Dietetic Association. Dietitian, Nutritionist, Nutritional Therapist or Diet Expert? A comprehensive guide to roles and functions. 2014.

136 Jennifer Sygo. Are 'superfoods' really that good for you? From kale to coconut water. The Independent. 25 August 2015.

137 Blair, Robert. (2012). Organic Production and Food Quality: A Down to Earth Analysis. Wiley-Blackwell, Oxford, UK. Pages 72, 223. ISBN 978-0-8138-1217-5

138 Alan D Dangour, Sakhi K Dodhia, Arabella Hayter, Elizabeth Allen, Karen Lock, and Ricardo Uauy. Nutritional quality of organic foods: a systematic review. Am J Clin Nutr September 2009 vol. 90 no. 3 680-685. 29 July 2009. 10.3945/ajcn.2009.28041

139 University of Missouri, "Organic milk finishes last in taste tests", http://foodscience.missouri.edu/news/organic-milk.php

Gluten-free diets

There is a condition called Coeliac disease (often spelt celiac) in which you are intolerant to gluten. If so, you should avoid it140.

Everyone else should be eating gluten. Foods with gluten in them are often highly nutritious141. Gluten-free alternatives are often stripped of these nutrients and contain higher levels of fat and sugar142, neither of which we usually lack.

Some people claim that you can develop gluten sensitivity without coeliac disease. This claim has not been proven143. In fact, most people who think they are gluten sensitive cannot tell the difference between eating gluten and gluten-free products144 and experience no symptoms145.

Branded diets

When I use the term "branded diets" I am talking about any diet with a specific name on it. For example the Atkins diet, or the paleo diet, both of which I will discuss here.

As a general rule, you should approach branded diets with caution. Some may be helpful, but most have little evidence to back them up and may not be an adequate substitute for properly planned and considered meals.

---

140 NHS Choices. Coeliac disease. 31 July 2014. http://www.nhs.uk/conditions/Coeliac-disease/Pages/Introduction.aspx

141 Rachael Rettner. Most People Shouldn't Eat Gluten-Free. Scientific American. 11 March 2013.

142 Siobhan Fenton. Gluten-free diets could be harmful for those who don't need them, expert warns. The Independent. 13 May 2016.

143 Jessica R Biesiekierski and Julie Iven. Non-coeliac gluten sensitivity: piecing the puzzle together. United European Gastroenterol J. 2015 Apr; 3(2): 160–165. doi: 10.1177/2050640615578388

144 Zanini, B., Baschè, R., Ferraresi, A., Ricci, C., Lanzarotto, F., Marullo, M., Villanacci, V., Hidalgo, A. and Lanzini, A. (2015), Randomised clinical study: gluten challenge induces symptom recurrence in only a minority of patients who meet clinical criteria for non-coeliac gluten sensitivity. Aliment Pharmacol Ther, 42: 968–976. doi:10.1111/apt.13372

145 Biesiekierski JR, Peters SL, Newnham ED, Rosella O, Muir JG, Gibson PR. No effects of gluten in patients with self-reported non-celiac gluten sensitivity after dietary reduction of fermentable, poorly absorbed, short-chain carbohydrates. Gastroenterology. 2013 Aug;145(2):320-8.e1-3. doi: 10.1053/j.gastro.2013.04.051. Epub 2013 May 4.

British Dietetic Association reviews

In 2016, the British Dietetic Association (BDA) reviewed 12 of the most popular diets to see if they were of any use146. I have summarised their findings below:

Diet	Conclusion
5:2 diet	Limited evidence for effectiveness. Fasting can be bad for your health. May help reduce calories.
Dukan diet	Unhealthy; lacks nutritional balance.
Paleo diet	Lacks variety, leading to nutritional deficiencies.
New Atkins diet	High levels of red meat and salt contradict current health advice.
Alkaline diet	The body does not need any help regulating its acidity levels.
Cambridge diet	Has side-effects. Eating so few calories can be dangerous to your health.
South Beach diet	Can cause nutritional deficiencies.
Slimming World diet	Sensible advice, but lacks education on calories and portion sizes.
Slim-Fast diet	Replacing food with Slim-Fast products does not help you make educated improvements to your diet.
LighterLife diet	Has side-effects. Eating so few calories can be dangerous to your health
WeightWatchers diet	Sensible advice.
Rosemary Conley diet	Sensible advice.

I will discuss general themes that appear here in the conclusion of this section.

Paleo diet

---

146 NHS Choices. Top diets review for 2016. 15 December 2014.
http://www.nhs.uk/Livewell/losewcight/Pages/top-10-most-popular-diets-review.aspx

The paleo diet is the most searched for diet on the internet147. Which is a shame, because as hypothesises go, this is probably one of the shakiest. Therefore, I am singling it out for special attention.

The concept is that the modern world is having us eat all kinds of crazy things and that this is bad. Instead, we should eat the same things that early humans ate because this was clearly better for us. Specifically, it focuses on the palaeolithic era, hence the name. Therefore it focuses on meat, fish, fruit and vegetables.

There are a number of problems with this thinking:

- It falls for the naturalistic fallacy: just because something is natural does not automatically make it good148
- We do not know what humans ate during the palaeolithic era149
- Our digestive abilities differ from those of our palaeolithic ancestors150
- Back in the "good old days" life expectancy was only a third of what it is today151 - in contrast, we live longer today in part because of the rich and varied diet we consume

On a theoretical level then, the paleo diet does not seem to make much sense.

On an evidence level, the picture is a little brighter. Some reviews suggest that the paleo diet could be helpful152. However, most agree that there is insufficient evidence to draw any conclusions153.

---

147 Niche Hacks. Niche Market Report – The Paleo Diet. 15 November 2016. http://nichehacks.com/wp-content/uploads/2013/12/NicheHacks-Paleo-Diet-Report.pdf

148 Naturalistic fallacy. Encyclopedia Britannica. 26 July 2012.

149 Peter S. Ungar, Mark F. Teaford. Human Diet: Its Origin and Evolution. 30 March 2002. ISBN: 0897897366

150 Marlene Zuk. Paleofantasy: What Evolution Really Tells Us about Sex, Diet, and How We Live. 3 February 2014. ISBN: 0393347923

151 Frederick L. Coolidge, Ph.D. and Thomas Wynn, Ph.D. The Truth About the Caveman Diet. Psychology Today. 22 November 2013. https://www.psychologytoday.com/blog/how-think-neandertal/201311/the-truth-about-the-caveman-diet

Summarising diet products

Many of the diets contain a mixture of helpful and unhelpful advice.

Nobody is arguing that a diet that focuses on fruits and vegetables, and away from processed foods, is anything but good for you. But the point is that any sensible advice on a balanced diet says this. You do not need some fad diet to give you this advice.

The diets that get the most favourable reviews are the ones that do not place restrictions on what you eat (because this reduces variety and thus leads to nutritional deficiencies) and provide education on calories and portion sizes.

The one possible use-case for such diets is if you struggle to follow general advice, and feel that a more structured and rule-based approach would help you stick to it. In which case, pick a diet that follows the above two rules of allowing you to maintain variety and providing evidenced-based education on healthy eating.

Another point to consider is sustainability. By this, I mean how long can you stick to it, rather than environmental sustainability. It is difficult to keep to diets with weird and wacky rules. Opting for improving our educational levels in the future is far more likely to produce long-term change.

Detox diets

Avoid detox diets.

The idea behind them is that toxins can build up in your body, and you can clear them out by using a special diet to *detox* your body. However, this simply is not true[154] nor is there any evidence detox diets work[155].

---

152 Eric W Manheimer, Esther J van Zuuren, Zbys Fedorowicz, and Hanno Pijl. Paleolithic nutrition for metabolic syndrome: systematic review and meta-analysis. Am J Clin Nutr October 2015 vol. 102 no. 4 922-932. doi: 10.3945/ajcn.115.113613

153 Pitt CE. Cutting through the Paleo hype: The evidence for the Palaeolithic diet. Aust Fam Physician. 2016 Jan-Feb;45(1):35-8.

154 The Truth About... Detox Diets. British Dietetic Association. 2006.

155 Klein AV, Kiat H. Detox diets for toxin elimination and weight management: a critical review of the evidence. J Hum Nutr Diet. 2015 Dec;28(6):675-86. doi: 10.1111/jhn.12286. Epub 2014 Dec 18.

This makes sense because your body is magnificent at cleaning up toxins. This is what your kidneys and liver are designed for. If they fail, and toxins do start building up, you can live *maybe* a couple of days. There is a reason people go to the hospital for dialysis three times a week. Assuming you have not died, you can safely move on with your life knowing that toxins are not building up in your body.

Eating disorders

The term *eating disorder* covers a variety of different conditions in which someone has an atypical relationship with food. This leads them changing their attitudes and behaviours, often resulting in unhealthy choices.

Eating disorders are more likely to occur in women than in men[156], and more likely to occur in young people than adults[157]. However, they can show up anywhere, particularly binge eating, that often shows up later in life.

Eating disorders are particularly relevant here because there is a strong correlation between eating disorders and anxiety[158].

Types of eating disorders

The most common types of eating disorders are:

Name	Description
Anorexia nervosa	Obsession with weight loss. You may starve yourself, experience an intense fear of weight gain and have self-esteem issues relating to your body.
Binge eating	Eating too much food over a short period. You may eat even when you are not hungry, and continue eating after you feel

---

156 James I. Hudson, Eva Hiripi, Harrison G. Pope, Jr., and Ronald C. Kessler. The Prevalence and Correlates of Eating Disorders in the National Comorbidity Survey Replication. Biol Psychiatry. 2007 Feb 1; 61(3): 348–358.

157 Swanson SA, Crow SJ, Le Grange D, Swendsen J, Merikangas KR. Prevalence and Correlates of Eating Disorders in Adolescents: Results From the National Comorbidity Survey Replication Adolescent Supplement. Arch Gen Psychiatry. 2011;68(7):714-723. doi:10.1001/archgenpsychiatry.2011.22.

158 National Collaborating Centre for Mental Health. Eating Disorders: Core interventions in the treatment and management of anorexia nervosa, bulimia nervosa and related eating disorders. 2004. ISBN: 1 85433 398 4

full. After, you may experience feelings of shame and guilt for having eaten so much.

Bulimia   Obsession with weight control. You may binge eat and then deliberately throw up to ensure you do not gain weight. You may experience self-esteem issues relating to your body.

Treatment for eating disorders

Eating disorders are typically treated using similar methods to anxiety. This may include cognitive behavioural therapy (CBT) and interpersonal psychotherapy. In some cases, it could include the use of antidepressants. Dietary counselling is also used.

If you think you have an eating disorder, the first step would be to speak to your GP. Or, if you feel uncomfortable doing that, there are a range of different charities and organisations that offer independent advice and assistance.

Cooking

There is a range of opinions about cooking. Some people love it, some people hate it, and some people are simply indifferent.

I am not sure I ever **hated** cooking, but I certainly used to think of it was a big waste of time. It was like brushing my teeth or getting dressed. I had to do, but I found it tedious as there were other things I wanted to be getting on with. If I could have eliminated it from my life with some nutrient pill, I would have taken it.

Now I feel the opposite. I love cooking. I find it therapeutic. This is most definitely a good thing because cooking is not going away anytime soon. We do not have the nutrient pill yet, so we have to prepare food in some manner, so if we can enjoy it, we are going to enjoy a much higher percentage of our lives.

Cooking is a form of self-care. Taking time out to prepare a healthy and nutritious meal for yourself (or occasionally an unhealthy and delicious meal) is as good for the soul as it is for the body. It is taking that time out, away from our worries, that is good for us.

For me, cooking is a form of mindfulness in itself. Sitting around meditating is hard to stick to every day. However, shutting off from the world and concentrating on a dish is much easier to do. You have to live in the moment when you are holding a very sharp knife.

Or, if I am not feeling particularly mindful on a certain evening, I will use the time to listen to some music or an audiobook. I cannot tell myself off for wasting time doing something frivolous like enjoying a good book because I am doing something necessary and productive at the same time.

So here is my pitch for why we should spend more time in the kitchen:

- You have to prepare food for yourself in some form or another. Cooking may take a little longer, but you would be spending some of that time microwaving meal anyway.
- Preparing meals yourself allows you to make them delicious.
- Preparing meals yourself makes it easier to hit your nutritional goals.
- Cooking gives you a sense of achievement when you complete a dish.
- Cooking is a great chance to give yourself permission to have some time off from the rest of the world.
- Cooking can be mindful.
- Developing your cooking skills is a form of lifelong learning, which we will discuss the benefits of in a later chapter.

Cooking for those who do not cook

If you would describe yourself as someone who "cannot cook" then cooking is probably **most** beneficial for you. It is a chance to learn a new skill and take some time out of your life that you otherwise would not do.

But where to start? Most cookbooks assume a level of proficiency already, and the many of the cookbooks that claim to be cookery courses may show you step-by-step how to use different techniques, but rarely hold you by the hand from step one.

Here are some resources that I recommend:

Jamie's Ministry of Food: If you are in the UK, Jamie's Ministry of Food is a great place to start. Here is the official blurb[159] from their website:

"I want to inspire you to get in the kitchen and cook meals for yourself and your family from scratch, whether you're a complete beginner or a good cook who likes simplicity. With some basic skills under your belt and a handful of recipes, you'll be able to prepare nutritious meals on any budget."

---

159 Jamie Oliver. Jamie's Ministry of Food. 11 January 2017.
http://www.jamieoliver.com/jamies-ministry-of-food/

I have friends who have undertaken their 8-week course and said they would highly recommend it. The prices are very reasonable.

The 4-Hour Chef: Tim Ferriss believes that anyone can become a master chef and makes that his aim in this book160. Whether or not that is the case, it does provide a sound introduction: it is deliberately laid out with simple recipes at the start that progressively becomes more involved.

Simple Cooking Channel: This YouTube channel has clocked up over a million subscribers161 thanks to its clear videos and easy-to-follow instructions. I still jump on one of Jason's videos every time I want to make honeycomb.

Cooking for the time poor

My argument for cooking, as with all of the aspects covered in this book, is that it is worth making time for it. We are all busy: what matters is what we prioritise. If we want to feel better, we need to prioritise our mind and body.

However, cooking does not have to take a long time. Often, it can be quicker to cook a meal from fresh than it can be to throw frozen food in the oven or order a takeaway.

Here are some options for cooking on a limited budget of time:

Stir-fry: When you stir-fry, you cook everything at a very high heat, so it is all done quickly. From start to finish you spend five minutes chopping vegetables, two minutes heating the wok and a final five minutes frying it all. Then you are done: just serve.

Slow cooking: A Slow cooker is a reasonably inexpensive addition to your kitchen and makes your life a whole lot easier. Put all the food in the cooker in the morning, set it for 8 hours and leave it. It will automatically turn off when done, and go into "keep warm" mode until you are ready to eat it. Pick up a copy of Heather Whinney's ***The Slow Cook Book***162, or just use the recipe cards including in your slow cooker.

---

160 Timothy Ferriss. The 4-Hour Chef: The Simple Path to Cooking Like a Pro, Learning Anything, and Living the Good Life. 2012. ISBN: 0547884591.

161 Simple Cooking Channel, https://www.youtube.com/user/SimpleCookingChannel

162 Heather Whinney. The Slow Cook Book. 1 September 2011. ISBN: 1405367822.

Recipe boxes: In recent years, a host of recipe box services have appeared. These include Hello Fresh and Gousto in the UK163, and Fresh Prep and Culiniste in Canada164. They supply you with pre-prepared boxes of ingredients, such as vegetables already portioned and pre-cut) and a recipe card for you to cook at home.

Chris's top five cookbook recommendations

I like to do things by the numbers. So, in 2016 I went through all of my cookbooks and measured how much I used each of them165. Doing this gave me an evidential basis for working out which cookbooks are the most useful.

In the list below, I use this data, along with a few other recommendations.

1. *River Cottage*. I will include all of Hugh Fearnley-Whittingstall's excellent River Cottage series in one item. Otherwise, it would just be a list of River Cottage books. My favourites are *Veg Every Day*166 and *River Cottage Every Day*167. However, I also enjoyed the *River Cottage Fish Book*168 and the *River Cottage Bread Handbook*169.

2. *Mary Berry*. The only other cookbooks that get anywhere near as much use as my River Cottage books are my two Mary Berry ones:

---

163 Kate Hilpern. 10 best recipe boxes. The Independent. 5 July 2015. http://www.independent.co.uk/extras/indybest/food-drink/best-recipe-boxes-kits-delivery-abel-and-cole-riverford-gousto-10364765.html

164 Brent Furdyk. 5 meal subscription services that will make your life easier. Global News. 4 April 2016. http://globalnews.ca/news/2616829/5-meal-subscription-services-that-will-make-your-life-easier/

165 Chris Worfolk. Which cookbooks are the most useful? Chris Worfolk's Blog. 24 September 2016. http://blog.chrisworfolk.com/2016/09/24/which-cookbooks-are-the-most-useful/

166 Hugh Fearnley-Whittingstall. River Cottage Veg Every Day! 19 September 2011. ISBN: 1408812126.

167 Hugh Fearnley-Whittingstall. River Cottage Every Day. 5 October 2009. ISBN: 0747598401.

168 Hugh Fearnley-Whittingstall, Nick Fisher. The River Cottage Fish Book. 19 November 2007. ISBN: 0747588694.

169 Daniel Stevens. The River Cottage Bread Handbook. 15 June 2010. ISBN: 158008186X.

*Mary Berry's Absolute Favourites*170 and *Mary Berry Cooks*171. Berry gives easy-to-follow instructions and almost always includes steps for doing things in advance and freezing for later use.

3. *Paul Hollywood's Bread*172. If you want to try your hand at bread making, this is an excellent place to start. There are so many different types of bread in this book.

4. *Michel Roux's Sauces*173. Not one for beginners, but an excellent book for improvers. You can build a meal around a sauce. Then just add whatever meat or vegetables Roux recommends.

5. *The 4-Hour Chef*174. See my explanation in the previous section.

Mindfulness in diet

Using mindful techniques is necessary for enjoying food more and ensuring we do not engage in too many unhealthy habits. Using mindfulness practice can turn mealtimes into a pleasure, where before they may have been a chore.

Mindful eating

Eating is something we have to do, so we may as well try to enjoy it. This sounds simple, but it is often something we forget to do. I have lost count of the times I have wolfed down a meal, not thinking about what I was putting in my body.

Not paying attention can lead to overeating. When we eat too fast, we are not paying attention to our stomachs. We do not know when to stop. In contrast, eating slowly can help us stop when we feel full175.

---

170 Mary Berry. Mary Berry's Absolute Favourites. 26 February 2015. ISBN: 1849908796.

171 Mary Berry. Mary Berry Cooks. 1 February 2014. ISBN: 1849906637.

172 Paul Hollywood. Paul Hollywood's Bread. 4 June 2013. ISBN: 1408840693.

173 Michel Roux. Sauces: Savoury And Sweet. 12 September 2011. ISBN: 1844006972.

174 Timothy Ferriss. The 4-Hour Chef: The Simple Path to Cooking Like a Pro, Learning Anything, and Living the Good Life. 2012. ISBN: 0547884591.

175 Bill Hendrick. Eating Slowly May Help Weight Control. WebMD Health News. 4 November 2009. http://www.webmd.com/diet/news/20091104/eating-slowly-may-help-weight-control

In contrast, paying attention allows you to really enjoy the food you eat. We are lucky enough to have the richest and most varied diet in human history176. Almost every fruit and vegetable is now permanently in season and available at a supermarket that only closes once per year. It's amazing!

It is so easy to let these experiences slip by. Biting into a juicy strawberry, smelling the aroma of an Indian curry or have a tender Argentinian beef fillet melt in your mouth. We miss how good they taste or what a miracle it is they are available on all our table at all.

Mindful meals

Here is an exercise: the next time you have a meal, slow down. Take your time. Enjoy every mouthful, or at very least, each new texture. Savour it on your tongue. How does it taste? How does it make you feel?

You might like the idea of this exercise. However, you might also be thinking "that sounds really stupid. What does it taste like? What are we, children?" If you do find yourself thinking that, that is a normal reaction to have. The exercise is still worth doing, though.

It **does** sound incredibly simple. And it is as an idea. However, implementing it is difficult. I am constantly reminding myself to do this, yet mealtime after mealtime I find myself slipping out of the present moment. You need to practice it. Even though it feels silly. It takes repetition.

Mindful treats

Using mindfulness when consuming treats such as chocolate, is nothing short of a superpower. Why? Because allows you to enjoy the chocolate more while eating less of it. Amazing, no? I have covered this on both the *Worfolk Anxiety Blog*177 and the *Worfolk Anxiety Podcast*178. I have reproduced it here:

---

176 Rob Lyons. Panic on a Plate: How Society Developed an Eating Disorder. 20 October 2011. ISBN: 1845402162.

177 Chris Worfolk. How to reduce unhealthy food with mindful eating. Worfolk Anxiety Blog. 12 December 2016. https://www.worfolkanxiety.com/blog/posts/how-to-reduce-unhealthy-food-with-mindful-eating

178 Chris Worfolk. How to eat less chocolate while enjoying it more. Worfolk Anxiety Podcast. 12 December 2016. https://www.worfolkanxiety.com/podcast/episodes/how-to-eat-less-chocolate-while-enjoying-it-more

Do you ever feel that you eat too much chocolate, sugar or other substances that are bad for you? Have you ever opened a snack, telling yourself you would only eat half of it, and then realised you had eaten the entire thing?

If you are like me, you may find yourself doing this on a regular basis.

I love chocolate. I love it! I have never tried heroin, but when people tell me about the rush they experience, I emphasise by thinking about the explosion of pure pleasure I experience when I bite into luxurious Belgian chocolate.

Sometimes I make pots of ganache. For the best experience, I have to use milk chocolate. Milk is always a winner. Dark chocolate I like too, but it depends on the situation. Some days I love it, some days I can leave it.

The one ganache I did not eat

Recently, I was eating one such chocolate pot, and stopped half way through. It occurred to me that I was not enjoying eating it. Yes, it was chocolatey, but I was not enjoying the bitterness on this particular day.

What would I normally do in this situation? I would keep eating it! Even though I was not enjoying it, and even though I was putting hundreds of kcals of fat and sugar into my body, I would just keep eating it.

But this time, I stopped eating and threw the rest away.

Why do we just keep eating?

Why is it that this is an unusual situation? Why is it that so often we just keep eating long after it has ceased to be pleasant? There are many reasons, and here are just some.

Fat and sugar give your brain a little hit of dopamine. Even though on a rational level we have decided we do not want any more dessert, our lower level functions want to keep taking that hit.

Second, we may be living with fixed expectations and rules. Have you ever noticed that most people finish the food on their plate, especially at restaurants? What are the odds that the amount of food on the plate happened to be exactly the amount of food the person wanted to eat?

The odds, of course, are small. But people just keep eating, long past being full because we have expectations that you "do not waste food" even though the additional food is of no use or advantage to your body. We feel an obligation to process it through our digestive system even at the detriment of our health, once it has been cooked.

So what do we do about it?

Conveniently, some of the techniques we can use to control anxiety can also be of use here.

First, eat mindfully. Eating can be a very pleasurable activity. But when our mind is all over the place, allowed to run around worrying about things, we lose this experience and fail to notice when we are not enjoying it. Eat in the moment and reap the rewards.

Second, spot the contradiction between how our lower and higher level brain functions are experiencing the situation. In anxiety, we might note "my higher reasoning says spiders are not harmful, but my lower brain is screaming to run". Spotting this, and recognising it as anxiety does not always help, but it does help us calm ourselves down.

Similarly, understanding why our body wants to keep eating, even though our higher brain has decided it is not enjoying the experience anymore, can help us make better choices.

Finally, fight against living my fixed rules. You do not have to finish a chocolate pot if you are not enjoying it. You are paying for every kcal you consume so make it count. Do not let social pressure dictate how you eat.

Okay, but what does this have to do with anxiety?

It connects to anxiety in two ways.

First, a good diet promotes good mental health. Healthy eating helps keep our mood stable, whereas cramming our body with junk food can contribute to low mood.

Second, by practising the skills we use in anxiety and applying it to our diet, it also strengthens the skills when we want to apply them to worries as well.

Mindful cooking

For me, cooking is one of the ultimate mindful activities. I struggle to sit down, cross my legs and allow thoughts to float through my mind like a cloud. However, ask me to concentrate on rustling up a dish, and I am your man.

It has a number of benefits:

•   It provides an activity to focus on when you are trying to live in the moment.

- It connects you with nature, when you handle ingredients, even if you will ultimately be *eating* that nature.
- It gives you sensory experiences to ground you in the moment. The cooking pot gives off smells. You have to taste it for seasoning. It crackles as you lay things on the grill. You see it transform before your eyes.
- It comes with a reward: a tasty and nutritious meal at the end. One that you will enjoy eating **and** will be good for you. Or, occasionally, one that will not be good for me, but that I will *really* enjoy eating.

Sometimes, it even throws in challenges. What happens when you have to stir a sauce for ten minutes, for example? This is a classic chance for your mind to wander. Will you be calm as the sky? Either way, it is a good chance to practice, with the knowledge that you will get back to knife-wielding around vegetables shortly after.

A mindful reminder

One of the reasons it is so difficult to practice mindful eating on a regular basis is that it is so easy to forget. Indeed, while writing this chapter, I ate my way through a chocolate bar without paying much attention.

If I can forget while writing a chapter about mindful eating, what hope have we got? Luckily, I have a few suggestions:

- Place a reminder on your kitchen table. One that you will notice when you sit down to eat.
- Write it on your hand.
- If you have lunch at the same time every day, set a reminder alarm on your phone.
- If you have breakfast from the same cereal box each day, write down a reminder and put it in the box.

A key to this is that it has to be *a little* unexpected. If you place a reminder on your kitchen table and leave it there for a few weeks, you may find you quickly start ignoring it. If this happens, it is time to change the reminder. Or, remove it for a few weeks, and then bring it back. Change this up. The brain notices novelty.

Summary

In this chapter, we learnt that diet has a significant and measurable effect on our mood. How we feel is directly affected by what we eat, drink and put into our bodies.

Diet is not something we can improve with fad detox programmes. We need to make sustainable changes, planning our meals in advance and recording and monitoring the things we want to change.

Mindfully eating can help us control our portion sizes and enjoy our food more.

Action steps

- Use the swaps list to provide some clean eating quick wins.
- Use a calorie tracking app if you are concerned about the amount you are eating.
- Use a journal or phone app to track your bad eating habits.
- Plan meals ahead to avoid resorting to unhealthy eating habits.
- Carry water around with you to remove barriers to hydration.
- Schedule time to cook.
- Practice mindful eating. Set yourself a reminder that you will see at mealtimes.

Sleep

Sleep is a challenging topic for many people with anxiety. Some of us find it difficult to get to sleep, and to stay asleep. Others find that they sleep too much. Both of these scenarios are normal for people with anxiety.

Why is sleep important?

A regular and healthy amount of sleep correlates with good physical health, good mental health, quality of life179 and productivity180. It affects a broad range of other aspects of our lives including our weight181.

Sleep affects our mood182. When your mood is low, lack of sleep will keep it depressed183.

What happens when we do not get enough sleep?

It is not just our physical health and mood that are affected by a lack of sleep. There are many other side-effects:

More pain. It is not entirely clear why sleep and pain are related, but there is a lot of evidence to suggest they are correlated184. Lack of sleep can maintain or increase chronic pain, joint pain and endogenous pain.

---

179 National Heart, Lung and Blood Institute. Why Is Sleep Important? 22 February 2012. https://www.nhlbi.nih.gov/health/health-topics/topics/sdd/why

180 MedlinePlus. The Importance of Sleep. National Institute of Health. Summer 2012 Issue: Volume 7 Number 2 Page 17.

181 Devon L. Golem, Jennifer T. Martin-Biggers, Mallory M. Koenings, Katherine Finn Davis, and Carol Byrd-Bredbenner. An Integrative Review of Sleep for Nutrition Professionals. Advances in Nutrition. November 2014 Adv Nutr vol. 5: 742-759, 2014. doi: 10.3945/an.114.006809

182 Zohar D, Tzischinsky O, Epstein R, Lavie P. The effects of sleep loss on medical residents' emotional reactions to work events: a cognitive-energy model. Sleep. 2005 Jan;28(1):47-54.

183 Mieke Sonnenschein, Marjolijn J. Sorbi, Lorenz J.P. van Doornen, Wilmar B. Schaufeli, Cora J.M. Maas. Evidence that impaired sleep recovery may complicate burnout improvement independently of depressive mood. Journal of Psychosomatic Research. April 2007 Volume 62, Issue 4, Pages 487-494. DOI: DOI: http://dx.doi.org/10.1016/j.jpsychores.2006.11.011

Impaired immune system. Sleep plays a major role in maintaining the immune system185, so if we do not get enough sleep, we are more likely to become ill186.

Impaired performance. Not sleeping enough impairs your apply to stay focused, short-term and long-term memory and your decision making abilities187. It reduces your performance, concentration and memory and reaction times188.

Difficulty at work. A study looking at sleep deprived doctors found that lack of sleep causes you to be more hostile to others, have more arguments with colleagues, make mistakes and take bad decisions189.

Greater risk of accidents. You are more likely to have an accident when you have not had enough sleep. Much of the research has focused on vehicle collisions190, but there is plenty of evidence that it affects other areas of life as well191.

---

184 Finan PH, Goodin BR, Smith MT. The association of sleep and pain: An update and a path forward. The journal of pain : official journal of the American Pain Society. 2013;14(12):1539-1552. doi:10.1016/j.jpain.2013.08.007.

185 Besedovsky L, Lange T, Born J. Sleep and immune function. Pflugers Archiv. 2012;463(1):121-137. doi:10.1007/s00424-011-1044-0.

186 Brown R, Pang G, Husband AJ, King MG. Suppression of immunity to influenza virus infection in the respiratory tract following sleep disturbance. Reg Immunol. 1989 Sep-Oct;2(5):321-5.

187 Alhola P, Polo-Kantola P. Sleep deprivation: Impact on cognitive performance. Neuropsychiatric Disease and Treatment. 2007;3(5):553-567.

188 Carskadon MA. Sleep in adolescents: the perfect storm. Pediatr Clin North Am. 2011 Jun;58(3):637-47. doi: 10.1016/j.pcl.2011.03.003.

189 Baldwin DC Jr, Daugherty SR. Sleep deprivation and fatigue in residency training: results of a national survey of first- and second-year residents. Sleep. 2004 Mar 15;27(2):217-23.

190 De Mello MT, Narciso FV, Tufik S, et al. Sleep Disorders as a Cause of Motor Vehicle Collisions. International Journal of Preventive Medicine. 2013;4(3):246-257.

191 Rogers AE. The Effects of Fatigue and Sleepiness on Nurse Performance and Patient Safety. In: Hughes RG, editor. Patient Safety and Quality: An Evidence-Based Handbook for Nurses. Rockville (MD): Agency for Healthcare Research and Quality (US); 2008 Apr. Chapter 40.

Why do we sleep?

This section is purely for those who want to geek out on the science of sleep. You do not need to know this information, so feel free to skip to the next section if that is not your thing.

Why exactly do we sleep, anyway?

The answer is not as obvious as you may thing. Sure, we all feel the **need** to sleep. But why? What benefit does it bring to us? It correlates with positive things, but what is the explanation for that?

For the moment, we do not know. A study published by PLOS Biology[192] concluded:

"While there is still no consensus on why animals need to sleep, it would seem that searching for a core function of sleep, particularly at the cellular level, remains a worthwhile exercise. Especially if, as argued here, sleep is universal, tightly regulated, and cannot be eliminated without deleterious consequences. In the end, the burden of proof rests with those who are attempting not only to reject the null hypothesis, but to gather positive evidence for the elusive phoenix of sleep."

In short, we need to sleep, but we do not know why.

A common misunderstanding is that we need to sleep to gain energy. This is not the case. We gain energy from consuming food, not from sleeping.

The philosopher, Daniel Dennett, has suggested that we make be looking at sleep the wrong way round. If instead, we ask "why do we wake up?", the question becomes a lot easier to answer.

If we take sleep as the default position, we then have to explain why we wake. This is easier to explain: we need to find food and procreate, both of which are hard to do while sleeping.

How much should we sleep?

The ideal amount of sleep is 7-9 hours per night[193].

---

192 Cirelli C, Tononi G (2008) Is Sleep Essential? PLoS Biol 6(8): e216. doi:10.1371/journal.pbio.0060216

Sleeping less than this on a regular basis is associated with a range of health problems including weight gain, heart disease, hypertension and depression.

There are some situations where it may be appropriate to sleep more than this. For example, if you are recovering from illness, catching up on sleep debt, or are a teenager, you genuinely do need a little more sleep (8-10 hours)194.

It is sometimes claimed that older people need less sleep than younger people. There is no evidence to support this claim. What there is evidence for is that older people find it harder to sleep195. Some have confused this with the *need* to sleep.

Your sleeping environment

The term sleeping environment refers to how you arrange and setup your bedroom. Creating a healthy sleep environment helps you get to sleep easier and stay asleep for longer.

Noise

Noise is important. Our body is constantly alert for it. Specifically, the amygdala is always listening out for it. If you remember back to the chapter on understanding anxiety, the amygdala is the part of the brain which likes to panic irrationally. This is not a beneficial combination.

The brain categorises noise levels as danger signals, which in turn creates stress hormones. That means that if you have a noisy bedroom, such as one where you can hear traffic or aeroplane noise all night, your brain may be becoming anxious even while you are asleep196.

---

193 Consensus Conference Panel, Watson NF, Badr MS, et al. Recommended Amount of Sleep for a Healthy Adult: A Joint Consensus Statement of the American Academy of Sleep Medicine and Sleep Research Society. Sleep. 2015;38(6):843-844. doi:10.5665/sleep.4716.

194 US National Sleep Foundation. Recommended sleep. 23 October 2016. https://sleepfoundation.org/sleep-topics/teens-and-sleep

195 Klerman EB, Dijk D-J. Age-related reduction in the maximal capacity for sleep - implications for insomnia. Current biology : CB. 2008;18(15):1118-1123. doi:10.1016/j.cub.2008.06.047.

196 Ising H, Kruppa B. Health effects caused by noise: Evidence in the literature from the past 25 years. Noise Health 2004;6:5-13

Evidence on whether you can improve the situation with earplugs is mixed. A 2010 study published in Critical Care suggested earplugs were beneficial to improving sleep quality197.

However, a 2015 Cochrane review of non-pharmacological interventions in hospitals concluded that most studies of using earplugs to improve sleep did not show positive results and that none of the studies that had been done were of high enough quality to draw firm conclusions198.

Light

The idea that light affects our quality of sleep and that we need it to be dark to sleep is a very intuitive one. Surprisingly, though, evidence to support the idea that we need darkness to sleep properly is not as abundant as you might expect.

Both studies I discussed in the section on noise also looked at whether sleep masks could improve sleep quality. Once again, opinion was divided. The NHS do not recommend reducing artificial light as a way to help you sleep better199.

However, we should not ignore the fact that many people simply prefer to sleep in the dark. If you are one of them, you may want to consider how dark your bedroom is. Some curtains, and blinds especially, do a poor job of blocking out light. So much so that "black-out blinds" are a whole separate category, as if that was not the job of regular blinds.

---

197 Hu R, Jiang X, Zeng Y, Chen X, Zhang Y. Effects of earplugs and eye masks on nocturnal sleep, melatonin and cortisol in a simulated intensive care unit environment. Critical Care. 2010;14(2):R66. doi:10.1186/cc8965.

198 Hu R, Jiang X, Chen J, Zeng Z, Chen XY, Li Y, Huining X, Evans DJW. Non-drug treatments for promoting sleep in adults in the intensive care unit. Cochrane. 6 October 2015.

199 NHS Choices. Do iPads and electric lights disturb sleep? 23 May 2013. http://www.nhs.uk/news/2013/05May/Pages/Do-iPads-and-electric-lights-disturb-sleep.aspx

Temperature

It is easier to sleep in a cool room than a warm one. This is because one of the stages of falling asleep is your body temperature dropping200. Doing this is easier to do when the room is cooler than it is when it is warmer.

Bed

For me, investing in a good mattress is money well spent. It is somewhere I am going to spend a third of my life, which is more time than I spend in my car, on my sofa, and almost as much time as I spend on my computer.

In a 2009 study found that a new mattress increased sleep quality and reduced back pain201. Specifically, the study looked at changing people's mattresses for medium-firm mattresses, though the evidence as to whether medium-firm mattresses are more suitable for relieving pain is unclear202.

The bedroom: a place to sleep

As we have discussed, a lot of sleep is about expectation. Therefore, we want to ensure that we associate our bedroom with sleep, and not a place where we do anything else.

Removing distractions

First, we want to make sure that the bedroom is not associated with other activities. This is not always possible. Sex for example typically happens in a bedroom, and it is inconvenient and unnecessary to relocate this to another room.

However, there is a lot of stimulation we can avoid in the bedroom. Your bedroom is not a place for watching TV, it is not your home-office, and it is

---

200 van den Heuvel CJ, Noone JT, Lushington K, Dawson D. Changes in sleepiness and body temperature precede nocturnal sleep onset: evidence from a polysomnographic study in young men. J Sleep Res. 1998 Sep;7(3):159-66.

201 Jacobson BH, Boolani A, Smith DB. Changes in back pain, sleep quality, and perceived stress after introduction of new bedding systems. Journal of Chiropractic Medicine. 2009;8(1):1-8. doi:10.1016/j.jcm.2008.09.002.

202 Mattresses for Chronic Back or Neck Pain: A Review of the Clinical Effectiveness and Guidelines. Canadian Agency for Drugs and Technologies in Health. 14 May 2014.

not your kitchen. Working or eating meals while in bed causes you to associate the bedroom with activities other than sleep203.

Note that we are talking about stimulation here, not distractions. For example, electric lights from phone chargers and other electronic devices are not considered stimulation. As we discussed in the section on light, there is no evidence that these reduce sleep quality204.

What happens when we work in bed

For many of us, work is a common cause of anxiety and frustration. What happens when we take this work to bed? We start building up an expectation that the bedroom is a place where we experience that anxiety and frustration.

When we go to bed, our mind is conditioned to think about work. Thoughts begin to race throughout mind. This is the exact opposite of what we want. We want our bodies conditioned to think of the bedroom as a place we go for a break from thinking and worrying.

Do not lie awake

As well as making the bedroom a distraction-free environment, we want to make it an insomnia-free environment. If you go to bed and just lie awake, you will condition yourself to expect that the bedroom is somewhere where you lie awake. Thus when you try to sleep, you will associate the bedroom with not being able to sleep and the cycle continues.

To break this cycle, we want to break this association. That means getting up and going somewhere else.

---

203 Richard R. Bootzin and Michael L. Perlis. Behavioral Treatments for Sleep Disorders. Chapter 2: Stimulus Control Therapy p21. DOI: 10.1016/B978-0-12-381522-4.00002-X

204 NHS Choices. Do iPads and electric lights disturb sleep? 23 May 2013. http://www.nhs.uk/news/2013/05May/Pages/Do-iPads-and-electric-lights-disturb-sleep.aspx

A sleep-friendly diet

Your diet affects the quality of sleep205. Whether it does this directly or because you find it easier to sleep when you have all the nutrients you need is unclear. There is no special "sleep food", except possibly milk.

It also works the other way. Having poor sleep can lead you to eat a poor diet206, so this can sometimes become a destructive cycle.

A study published by the British Medical Journal found an improvement in sleep quality based on avoiding certain substances before going to bed207.

What to avoid	When to avoid it
Caffeine	After noon
Alcohol	Two hours before going to bed
Nicotine	Two hours before going to bed
Heavy meals	Two hours before going to bed

A sleep friendly routine

There are specific behaviours you can practice that will help you sleep better.

Have a regular bedtime

The body is a creature of habit so once you get it into a routine, it will find it easier to follow. Therefore if you can go to bed and get up at the same time every day, you may find it easier to sleep.

Take a warm bath before bed

Taking a warm (not hot) bath can increase the amount of REM sleep that you get208. The theory behind this is that falling asleep is accompanied by

205 Katri Peuhkuri, Nora Sihvola, Riitta Korpela. Diet promotes sleep duration and quality. Nutrition Research 32 (2012) 309 – 319.

206 Chaput JP. Sleep patterns, diet quality and energy balance. Physiol Behav. 2014 Jul;134:86-91. doi: 10.1016/j.physbeh.2013.09.006. Epub 2013 Sep 17. DOI: 10.1016/j.physbeh.2013.09.006

207 Lichstein KL, Wilson NM, Johnson CT. Stimulus control combined with relaxation improved sleep in secondary insomnia. Evid Based Mental Health 2000;3:116 doi:10.1136/ebmh.3.4.116

a drop in body temperature. Therefore if you put your body in a warm bath for a while, and then take it out, your body will read this is a cue for falling asleep.

Trouble sleeping

It is difficult, often impossible, to sleep when you have thoughts racing through your head. This is an issue because many people with anxiety find that their mind is running at full speed twenty-four seven.

Expectation of sleep

Have you ever lay awake stressing about how you need to fall asleep as soon as possible because you have to be up early the next day? Did that make it easier to sleep, or more difficult?

My money is that you found it was the latter. When we worry about the need to fall asleep, that increases our anxiety, which makes it harder to get sleep.

We can represent this on a diagram. You might find this pattern rather familiar by now because so often with anxiety, we find ourselves in cycles.

208 Wen-Chun Liao, RN, PhD, Assistant professor, Ming-Jang Chiu, MD, PhD, Visiting staff, Associate professor, and Carol A. Landis, RN, DNSc, FAAN, Professor. A Warm Footbath before Bedtime and Sleep in Older Taiwanese with Sleep Disturbance. Res Nurs Health. Author manuscript; available in PMC 2009 Oct 1. DOI: 10.1002/nur.20283

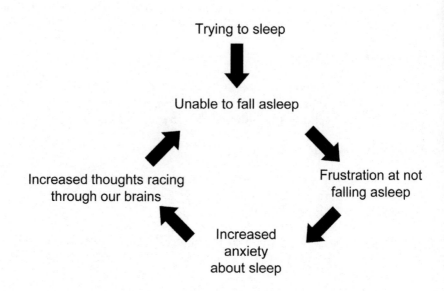

Trying to sleep

Unable to fall asleep

Frustration at not falling asleep

Increased anxiety about sleep

Increased thoughts racing through our brains

What this tells us is that the ability to fall asleep has a lot to do with our expectations of sleep. The relationship is inverse: if you expect to be able to sleep and become frustrated, you will find it hard to sleep, whereas if you relax and do not try and fall asleep you are more likely to.

What is insomnia?

Insomnia is an inability to get to sleep or stay asleep for long enough. Insomnia could express itself in several ways:

- Not being able to fall asleep
- Finding yourself laying awake for long periods
- Waking up several times in the night
- Waking up early in the morning and being unable to get back to sleep

Insomnia is common, especially in older people, with estimates of prevalence suggesting it affects between 6% and 30% of the population209.

---

209 Roth T. Insomnia: Definition, Prevalence, Etiology, and Consequences. Journal of Clinical Sleep Medicine : JCSM : official publication of the American Academy of Sleep Medicine. 2007;3(5 Suppl):S7-S10.

Insomnia and anxiety

Insomnia and anxiety often come hand-in-hand210. Suffering from anxiety makes you more likely to suffer from insomnia in the future. Similarly, suffering from insomnia makes you more likely to suffer from anxiety in the future.

Treating insomnia can reduce symptoms of anxiety211.

Treatment for insomnia

Insomnia is treatable, so you should speak to your GP if you are experiencing problems. The first thing they will suggest is looking at your sleep environment and what lifestyle changes you can make, just as we are discussing here.

There are also further treatments which I have discussed below.

Sleeping tablets

I will not discuss sleeping tablets in too much detail. After all, this book is about designing a lifestyle so that you do not have to use medication! However, I think it is important to know what the options are if you need them.

Sleeping tablets can be tricky beasts because they raise your expectations of sleep. As we have already discussed, expecting to be able to can be a cause of sleeplessness, so if sleeping tablets help build up these expectations, they could potentially do harm as well as good.

Tablets can only do so much. If you think about holding a human body unconscious against its will, that is serious business. You are basically talking about a general anaesthetic, which is only administered in a hospital. In comparison, sleeping tablets can only help the body do what it would do anyway.

On a positive note, the clinic term for sleeping tablets is "hypnotics", which is a pretty cool.

---

210 Markus Jansson-Fröjmark, Karin Lindblom. A bidirectional relationship between anxiety and depression, and insomnia? A prospective study in the general population. Journal of Psychosomatic Research 64 (2008) 443–449.

211 Staner L. Sleep and anxiety disorders. Dialogues in Clinical Neuroscience. 2003;5(3):249-258.

Sleeping tablets should only be used in the short term because they cause side effects and you can become dependent on them. They do not tackle the underlying reason for the insomnia so need to be used in conjunction with other treatments.

However, they can be useful if they are effective because they help you break the cycle of thinking you cannot sleep, worrying about it and thus keeping yourself awake. Short-term usage can make it easier to sleep and therefore reinforce the idea that you can fall asleep once you stop taking the pills.

You can by sleeping tablets over the counter (known as OTC sleeping tablets). However, there is little evidence that these are effective[212]. Many are antihistamines re-purposed because they make people drowsy. These can cause the same side effects as you experience with insomnia itself[213].

Prescription sleeping tablets

If you doctor prescribes you a sleeping tablets, it will probably be from one of three categories.

Benzodiazepines are drugs which relax you. There are several types, but perhaps the most well known is *diazepam*, initially marketed as *valium*[214]. They make you feel more relaxed, reduce anxiety and promote sleep.

Official guidelines state that benzodiazepines should not be used long-term because they have a long list of side effects, become less effective over

---

212 Jill U. Adams. Over-the-counter sleep aids: The research on their effectiveness is limited, experts say. The Washington Post. 25 November 2015.

213 Pagel JF, Parnes BL. Medications for the Treatment of Sleep Disorders: An Overview. Primary Care Companion to The Journal of Clinical Psychiatry. 2001;3(3):118-125.

214 Diazepam. Drugs.com. 24 October 2016. https://www.drugs.com/diazepam.html

time215 and are addictive216. Despite this, some doctors do prescribe them long-term217.

Z-drugs are similar to benzodiazepines in terms of effects and side-effects. However, they are chemically different, and therefore also known as *nonbenzodiazepines*.

Perhaps the most well-known brand is *zopiclone*. They all pretty much do the same thing, so if one does not work there is no point trying the others218.

Circadin is a medication specifically for older people (people over the age of 55). As we age, we find it harder to regular our sleep cycle219. Circadin contains a hormone known as *melatonin* which is responsible for helping to regulate this cycle. This seems to be effective in helping people with some sleep disorders, but not insomnia220.

CBT-I

Cognitive Behavioural Therapy for Insomnia, known as CBT-I, is a special form of cognitive behavioural therapy specifically designed to help people with insomnia.

There are several components to CBT-I:

---

215 Longo LP, Johnson B. Addiction: Part I. Benzodiazepines--side effects, abuse risk and alternatives. Am Fam Physician. 2000 Apr 1;61(7):2121-8.

216 Richard C. Oude Voshaar, Jaap E. Couvée, Anton J. L. M. Van Balkom, Paul G. H. Mulder, Frans G. Zitman. Strategies for discontinuing long-term benzodiazepine use. The British Journal of Psychiatry Sep 2006, 189 (3) 213-220; DOI: 10.1192/bjp.189.3.213

217 Tauseef Mehdi. Benzodiazepines Revisited. Benzodiazepines Revisited. Benzodiazepines Revisited.

218 National Institute for Health and Clinical Excellence. Guidance on the use of zaleplon, zolpidem and zopiclone for the short-term management of insomnia. 28 April 2004.

219 C.A Czeisler, MD, M Dumont, PhD, J.F Duffy, MBA, J.D Steinberg, MD, G.S Richardson, MD, E.N Brown, MD, R Sánchez, AB, C.D Ríos, MD, J.M Ronda, MS. Association of sleep-wake habits in older people with changes in output of circadian pacemaker. The Lancet. Volume 340, Issue 8825, 17 October 1992, Pages 933-936. DOI: 10.1016/0140-6736(92)92817-Y

220 Buscemi N, Vandermeer B, Pandya R, et al. Melatonin for Treatment of Sleep Disorders: Summary. 2004 Nov. In: AHRQ Evidence Report Summaries. Rockville (MD): Agency for Healthcare Research and Quality (US); 1998-2005. 108.

Sleep restriction therapy. This involves deliberately keeping yourself awake so that you only sleep at the time you would typically fall asleep anyway. The idea is that you stay up and only give yourself the amount of sleep you are already getting, and then gradually bring bedtime forward.

For example, let's say that you are always lying awake until 3 am, even though you try and sleep from 11 pm to 7 am. With sleep restriction therapy you would force yourself to stay up until 3 am, and then have your four hours sleep. Once this is established, you would gradually move your 3 am bedtime forward until you reached 11 pm.

Whether sleep restriction therapy works is not clear. There is some evidence that it improves sleep time[221]. However, other studies have suggested it reduces sleep time and causes increased sleepiness during the day[222].

Stimulus control is about making the bedroom be associated with sleep. That means removing all stimulation from the room, such as TVs or other distractions. It also means that if you are unable to fall asleep within a set period, typically ten minutes, you have to get up and do thing else. The idea is to break the connection of the bedroom being somewhere where you lie awake.

Sleep hygiene is about educating yourself on good things to do to aid sleep. For example, you should avoid heavy meals before you go to bed, but you should use relaxing activities, such as taking a bath.

Relaxation training provides you with a set of techniques to help you relax. The idea is that if you can practice being more relaxed before going to bed, you will find it easier to drift off.

Be kind to your sleepy self

If you do find that you are unable to sleep, it is easy to become self-critical and start beating yourself up. Instead, I would encourage you to be kind to

---

221 Miller CB, Espie CA, Epstein DR, Friedman L, Morin CM, Pigeon WR, Spielman AJ, Kyle SD. The evidence base of sleep restriction therapy for treating insomnia disorder. Sleep Med Rev. 2014 Oct;18(5):415-24. doi: 10.1016/j.smrv.2014.01.006. Epub 2014 Feb 12.

222 Kyle SD, Miller CB, Rogers Z, Siriwardena AN, Macmahon KM, Espie CA. Sleep restriction therapy for insomnia is associated with reduced objective total sleep time, increased daytime somnolence, and objectively impaired vigilance: implications for the clinical management of insomnia disorder. Sleep. 2014 Feb 1;37(2):229-37. doi: 10.5665/sleep.3386.

yourself. Not only will it make your life more pleasant, but in the long term, it will also make it easier to sleep.

Enjoying your insomnia

Many people with anxiety dread going to bed. They cannot sleep and know that they are unlikely to sleep, so going through the struggle of trying to fall asleep every night becomes an unpleasant chore. This is unfortunate because the negative thoughts mean you are less likely to be able to drift off.

Instead, we want to relax and go easy on ourselves. One way to do this is to go on a mission to enjoy your insomnia.

It may have been suggested to you that if you cannot sleep, you should get up and do some housework. This is fine if you enjoy chores, but most of us do not.

Instead, why not do something fun? Is there a TV show that everyone is talking about but that you have never found time to watch? What a perfect time to binge-watch the entire series. Or perhaps you play video games or like to read, but often do not because there are so many other distractions and jobs to be done in life.

Bedtime is your time. Therefore, if you cannot sleep and get up to spend a night playing video games because you cannot sleep, nobody can blame you for that. You can spend the time guilt-free knowing that relaxing is exactly what you **should** be doing at this point.

Nor should you feel guilty that you **should** be "trying to sleep". Worrying about it will make you less likely to sleep, whereas relaxing and enjoying yourself will make it more likely.

Phone in sick

It is easy to get caught up in a thought cycle like this:

"I need to sleep because I have to be up for work in 5 hours." "I need to sleep because I have to be up for work in 3 hours." "I need to sleep because I have to be up for work in 2 hours."

On and on it goes for hours. You are trapped in a thought pattern of stressing that you will not get enough sleep before you have to get up the next morning for an appointment, to go to work, or any other commitments you have.

If you were up all night vomiting, you would probably phone in sick.

However, with insomnia, despite the fact that we often feel just as bad, we feel it is our fault that this has happened. We treat ourselves like we have a self-induced hangover and refuse to give ourselves the time off to recover.

This is nonsense. If you find that you have lost an entire night's sleep and feel terrible in the morning, remind yourself that it is not your fault and if appropriate, phone in sick.

Ideas for getting to sleep

If you are struggling to fall asleep, I have provided a few suggestions here.

Write down thoughts and ideas

If I get a thought in my head or have something to remember, trying to sleep is a waste of time. It goes round and round in my mind because my mind is paranoid that if I fall asleep, I will forget about an idea that it has deemed essential.

The way out of this cycle is to write it down. Making a note of it tells your mind that you have not forgotten about it and will get back to it later.

You can also try this for any anxious thoughts you are having. This helps clarify to yourself what you are worrying about it and helps you to relax, knowing that you are not going to *forget* to think about whatever is worrying you later.

Think about something else

One of the biggest enemies of sleep for the anxious is that our minds are constantly racing around. There is no "off" button, so when we want to turn off the thoughts and sleep, we find we cannot.

How do I cope with this? I don't even try.

I cannot turn the thoughts in my mind off, so I redirect them instead. I have my personal daydream world that I sent my mind to when it is time to sleep. Rather than clearing my mind, I send it to think about something else.

This way, my mind can continue to run at a million miles an hour, but in a scenario of my choosing. Rather than focusing on all the worries I have, it is free to play in a world of my creation, where I have control over what happens.

I do not go into details about it, but it is a world roughly based on reality, except when that becomes inconvenient, and has a lot of quite detailed characters. Think of it as a cartoon where you can just reset the plot every night and have a new adventure.

This one is from my personal vault of experiences. I will not claim it is backed up by any studies that I know of. It is not even something I developed consciously; it evolved over the past few decades as an emergent technique for helping myself sleep.

However, the idea of redirecting our attention rather than trying to clear our mind can be useful. This technique is used in mindfulness practice to improve focus223.

Should you try counting sheep?

The iconic image of someone trying to fall asleep is probably a cartoon of someone lying in bed counting as sheep jump over a fence. It is not clear why. There does not seem to be any evidence that this is helpful.

However, a study by Oxford University suggested that doing a mentally strenuous activity could help you fall asleep simply by distracting your mind with mental imagery224.

Specifically, the study suggested that you need to distract yourself with a visualisation exercise, rather than merely general distraction.

A daydream might work for this: maybe there is hope for my theory after all.

The same old film script

Another suggestion from my personal vaults of experience is to watch the same film over and over again. I use this one especially when I am ill (or health anxiety makes me think I am ill!) to help me calm down and drift off.

Pick a film and watch it every night when you go to bed. If you find that you are waking up several times in the night you may want to set it to loop so that when you wake up, you find the same film playing.

---

223 Focus and mindfulness meditation. Headspace. 27 October 2016.

224 Harvey AG, Payne S. The management of unwanted pre-sleep thoughts in insomnia: distraction with imagery versus general distraction. Behav Res Ther. 2002 Mar;40(3):267-77.

The theory behind this is that you come to associate the film with sleep and therefore condition your body that when the film comes on, it is time to sleep.

It has to be a film you know well. That way you will know what is going to happen next. If not, you will get caught up in actually watching the film, wanting to find out what will happen next, and this will make you more alert.

Sleeping for parents

If you have young children, you might be thinking "this is all very well, but there is no much I can do about my children waking me up." This is true, having children can be incredibly difficult.

However, where possible, there is a balancing act. Sleep deprivation decreases your ability to parent during the day[225].

When my daughter cries in the middle of the night, I comfort her. However, if she is still crying an hour later, I go back to bed. Yes, I know, I am a terrible parent (during the night). But, I am a better parent during the day.

Biphasic sleeping

Biphasic sleeping is the idea of breaking your sleep into two parts. There is also polyphasic sleeping which involves breaking your sleep into even more chunks.

There is evidence that humans have historically used biphasic sleep[226]. However, there is no evidence it is more beneficial than monophasic sleep.

What about napping?

If you are struggling with insomnia, naps are not a good idea. Napping can increase the symptoms[227].

---

225 Meltzer, Lisa J.; Mindell, Jodi A. Relationship between child sleep disturbances and maternal sleep, mood, and parenting stress: A pilot study. Journal of Family Psychology, Vol 21(1), Mar 2007, 67-73. http://dx.doi.org/10.1037/0893-3200.21.1.67

226 Stephanie Hegarty. The myth of the eight-hour sleep. BBC World Service. http://www.bbc.co.uk/news/magazine-16964783

Nor is napping recommended for young children. A study of 3-5-year-olds found that those who napped slept less at night, performed less well in tests and did less well in education228.

For everyone else, you should limit napping to no more than 30 minutes at a time229. Any longer, and you may reach deep sleep. This can lead to you feeling **more tired** when you wake up half way through a sleep cycle.

Sleep diaries

We have already talked about the important of writing things down to give us a firm evidence base when making decisions. Keeping a sleep diary helps you track the sleep you are getting and what affects it. This allows you to identify patterns and implement changes to improve your sleep.

You can find pre-printed sleep diaries online, or you can make you own. A good sleep diary will ask you:

• What time did you go to bed?
• How long did it take you to fall asleep? (Obviously, this is an estimate)
• How many times did you wake up during the night?
• What time did you wake up?
• What time did you get out of bed?
• How do you feel this morning?
• How would you rate your quality of sleep last night on a 1-10 scale?

This in itself allows you to measure how well you are doing and if there are any patterns between your bed time and your sleep. However, to make it more useful, you could also ask yourself the following questions before going to bed:

• Did I take a nap today?
• Did I do any exercise today?

---

227 Mayo Clinic, "Napping: Do's and don'ts for healthy adults", http://www.mayoclinic.org/healthy-lifestyle/adult-health/in-depth/napping/art-20048319

228 Lam JC, Mahone EM, Mason TBA, Scharf SM. The Effects of Napping on Cognitive Function in Preschoolers. Journal of developmental and behavioral pediatrics : JDBP. 2011;32(2):90-97. doi:10.1097/DBP.0b013e318207ecc7.

229 Michael Breus. Napping Tips: 7 Expert Strategies For Maximizing Your Naptime. Huffington Post. 28 May 2013. http://www.huffingtonpost.com/2013/05/28/napping-tips-expert-strat_n_3320571.html

- What did I eat today? When was my last meal?
- What did I drink today? When did I last have a caffeinated drink? Did I drink alcohol?
- What was my routine before going to bed?

Asking these questions allows you to spot patterns in your lifestyle, and how they affect your sleep. However, it is also a lot to fill in every day. Try doing it for 30 days. You can do it for just 30 days, right? Then look for patterns and see what you can improve.

Mindfulness and sleep

Mindfulness is unlikely to form a large part of your sleep behaviour because you are supposed to be, well, asleep. However, there are a few mindfulness practices that can be applied.

If you find yourself laying awake, and frustrated that you cannot fall asleep, this is a good opportunity to be kind to yourself and allow those thoughts to come and go. Every time you feel "I must fall asleep" or "I am angry that I cannot fall asleep", try to let the thought wash over you. Imagine it as a wave that washes over you and then retreats to the sea. Giving it attention will not help you sleep.

There is also evidence that mindfulness meditation during the day can improve your sleep[230]. Therefore, if sleep is a particular problem for you, you may wish to invest some time practising mindfulness skills during the day.

Summary

In this chapter, we learnt that getting enough sleep has a positive effect on your mood. In contrast, lack of sleep correlates with poor physical and mental health, impaired performance and a greater risk of accidents.

There are lots of things we can do to improve our sleep, from designing a better sleep environment to implementing a regular bedtime routine.

---

230 David S. Black, PhD, MPH; Gillian A. O'Reilly, BS1; Richard Olmstead, PhD2; et al. Mindfulness Meditation and Improvement in Sleep Quality and Daytime Impairment Among Older Adults With Sleep Disturbances. JAMA Intern Med. 2015;175(4):494-501. doi:10.1001/jamainternmed.2014.8081

Action steps

- Use a sleep diary to track your sleep. Are you getting 7-9 hours per night?
- Decide on a regular bedtime and stick to it.
- Work backwards: no meals, alcohol or nicotine two hours before this time. Make it a rule for yourself.
- Can you set yourself a rule for the last time you will have caffeine? Ideally noon, but you could start at 6 pm and gradually move it forwards.
- Review your sleep environment and make changes. Can you reduce noise? Remove distractions?

Relaxation

Relaxation is not about crossing your legs and slipping into a deep state of zen. Feel free to do that if you enjoy it, but it does little for me. This is about injecting some fun into your life. Give yourself permission to take some time off from worrying. This is often referred to as self-love.

Doing this is not easy. I regularly spend time beating myself up. Usually in a psychological sense. Sometimes in a physical sense (such as running a half marathon). However, relaxation is an enjoyable thing to do.

Why spend time relaxing?

It may be obvious why you should relax. But, even so, many of us do not spend the time we should. Perhaps because we do not believe that we should. I will deal with that later in this chapter. First, I think we should remind ourselves why relaxing is a good thing to do.

It is a fun thing to do

Having fun is fun. That is a tautology. However, when you have so much anxiety in your life, it is easy to forget that there used to be a real pleasure in doing things. There still can be: but we have to work for it.

By work, I mean get over the little voice in your head that tells you that should be doing something else. I like to watch NFL. However, to get the most out of it, I need to concentrate on the game. The temptation to open my laptop and do some work is high. We must resist.

When I do resist, I have a much more pleasant evening. I have an enjoyable evening. One in which I spent my time in a pleasing manner. It is wonderful to re-discover that feeling.

It builds your mental strength

You only have so much willpower per day[231]. Therefore, if you have a list of high resistance tasks and low resistance tasks, you should make sure you

---

231 Baumeister, et al. (1998). Ego depletion: is the active self a limited resource? Journal of Personality and Social Psychology, 74, 1252-1265.

do the high resistance tasks first, or by the end of the day, there is no way you will have the willpower left.

"If it's your job to eat a frog, it's best to do it first thing in the morning. And If it's your job to eat two frogs, it's best to eat the biggest one first." Unknown, but commonly attributed to Mark Twain.

Another way to put it is that willpower is like a muscle. Using it will make it stronger in the long term. But, in the short term, we need to rest it to give it time to recover.

How do we rebuild this strength, shake off the tiredness we feel and increase our mood? We relax232. It is the magic ingredient that allows us to face the world again.

IF YOUR JOB IS TO

EAT A FROG

IT IS BEST TO DO IT

FIRST THING

IN THE MORNING

---

232 Tice, D., et al. (2007). Restoring the self: positive affect helps improve self-regulation following ego depletion. Journal of Experimental Social Psychology, 43, 379-384. DOI: http://dx.doi.org/10.1016/j.jesp.2006.05.007

It helps you learn more and develop skills

When you are not engaging in a highly taxing task, the brain is anything but inactive. It is processing information, developing skills and consolidating knowledge: arguably it is only at this later point when learning occurs233. Even developing things like our social skills may occur, in part, when we are giving our brain "a rest"234.

Relaxation combats the negative effects of stress

Stress causes the release of a hormone named cortisol. Having high levels of cortisol is associated with a number of problems, including:

- Increased risk of having a stroke235
- Increased risk of heart disease236
- Increased risk of depression237
- Poor decision making238

Spending time relaxing can reduce cortisol levels239. Spending time relaxing is like exercising and eating well: it is an essential part of a healthy lifestyle.

---

233 Ferris Jabr. Why Your Brain Needs More Downtime. Scientific American. 15 October 2013. https://www.scientificamerican.com/article/mental-downtime/

234 Mary Helen Immordino-Yang, Joanna A. Christodoulou, Vanessa Singh. Rest Is Not Idleness: Implications of the Brain's Default Mode for Human Development and Education. Perspectives on Psychological Science. Vol 7, Issue 4, 2012.

235 Amanda Chan. Work Stress Could Raise Stroke Risk: Study. Huffington Post. 27 December 2011. http://www.huffingtonpost.com/2011/12/27/work-stress-stroke-risk-job-_n_1158897.html

236 Judith A Whitworth, Paula M Williamson, George Mangos, and John J Kelly. Cardiovascular Consequences of Cortisol Excess. Vasc Health Risk Manag. 2005 Dec; 1(4): 291–299.

237 Maia Szalavitz. Study: How Chronic Stress Can Lead to Depression. Time Magazine. 3 August 2011. http://healthland.time.com/2011/08/03/study-how-chronic-stress-can-lead-to-depression/

238 M. Mather, N. R. Lighthall. Risk and Reward Are Processed Differently in Decisions Made Under Stress. Current Directions in Psychological Science, 2012; 21 (1): 36 DOI: 10.1177/0963721411429452

Should statements

When looking at *negative automatic thoughts*, we spend time looking for "should statements". These are negative thoughts we give ourselves about expectations: "I should be able to do this" or "I should not feel this way".

I want to replace them with a different set. Here are some should statements that are more positive:

1. You should be okay with feeling some anxiety from time to time. It is not a crime.
2. You should give yourself permission to relax and unwind. Allowing yourself some "me time" is essential to maintaining a healthy mind.
3. You should allow yourself to be unproductive. You do not have to be going at full speed constantly.
4. You should look after your needs. Other people's needs are important too, but there has to be a balance.
5. You should resist feeling guilty when you do something you enjoy. You only get one life and should be allowed to enjoy it.

Giving yourself permission

The first step to relaxing is allowing yourself to relax. This point might sound obvious, but so many of us fail to do it. We feel that we cannot waste a single second: that every moment we must be doing something meaningful and productive.

This idea misses an important point: relaxing *is* meaningful and productive. It is not just recharging your batteries. It is giving yourself time to enjoy life and grow physically and emotionally.

Recovery miles

When professional athletes train for a long distance race, they do interval training sessions. This involves a cycle of working hard, then slowing down for a bit, and repeating this cycle over and over. It is tough.

---

239 Jones D, Owens M, Kumar M, Cook R, Weiss SM. The effect of relaxation interventions on cortisol levels in HIV-seropositive women. J Int Assoc Provid AIDS Care. 2014 Jul-Aug;13(4):318-23. DOI: 10.1177/2325957413488186

After the training session, they will do a recovery run. At first glance, this might seem like unproductive time. They are just going easy on their body before they can go on with the hard training.

But this is not the case. It turns out that the recovery run is essential to improving your body.

The way to run faster is to overload your body and then allow it to adapt. However, the body does not adapt well when it is under stress. It is only after, during the recovery run, when the adaptation happens[240].

Similarly, allowing your mind to relax is not just about resting it until it can "go again". It is about allowing yourself to grow and improve as a person. This growth happens occurs when you give your mind some time off.

Objections to relaxing

Even if we can convince ourselves that relaxing might be a good idea, there is usually a list of reasons why it is also a bad one. In this section, I will explain why many of these reasons do not hold water.

I will not enjoy it

Does this sound familiar: "I could do that thing I used to like, but I will just spend the whole time worrying. So I won't enjoy it, so there is no point doing it."?

If so, I have news for you: relaxing takes work. It is a skill. Like mindfulness meditation, or playing the tuba, you need to develop your relaxation powers. Fun is not always out-of-the-box fun for those with anxiety. We need to put some effort in and focus on enjoying ourselves. Just like I have to practice not picking up the laptop when I am watching NFL.

I feel guilty

See above.

I do not have time

In life, there is always an endless list of things to do. Even if we are not procrastinating, or doing genuine chores, we can often feel like we need to

---

240 Owen Barder. Easy runs & rest. Running For Fitness. 5 January 2017.
http://www.runningforfitness.org/book/chapter-9-the-training-cookbook/easy-runs-rest

spend time on bigger things, like "sorting out" our life or working towards our future.

I used to tell myself "if you want to be a real winner, you need to work hard. Use every minute you have." However, this does not map to what successful people do.

Steve Jobs, co-founder of **Apple Computers**, died with a net worth of $19 billion. He spent summers chasing down old Bob Dylan records and living on a fruit farm.

Richard Branson, the founder of **Virgin**, has a net worth of $5 billion. He spent years breaking the world record for crossing the Atlantic by boat and trying to fly around the world in a hot air balloon.

Jeff Bezos (**Amazon**, £67 billion) drives his children to school every morning[241]. Mark Zuckerberg (**Facebook**, $50 billion) learnt to speak Mandarin[242]. Jim Clark (**Netscape**, $2 billion) seems to spend **most** of his time building remote-controlled yachts[243].

It is not true that successful people devote their entire lives to work. On the contrary, they focus when they are at work and when they are not at work, they relax and do other things.

How to relax

Forgive me for using yet another patronising title. You probably know how to relax, just like you knew you **should** relax. However, so often we do not do it, so it is worth us chanting the mantra over and over again to help reinforce those beliefs.

Let's recap as to how exactly we spend time relaxing.

241 Brad Stone. The Everything Store: Jeff Bezos and the Age of Amazon. 15 October 2013. ISBN: 0316219266

242 Malcolm Moore. How good really is Mark Zuckerberg's Mandarin? The Telegraph. 24 October 2014. http://www.telegraph.co.uk/technology/mark-zuckerberg/11182575/How-good-really-is-Mark-Zuckerbergs-Mandarin.html

243 Michael Lewis. The New New Thing: A Silicon Valley Story. 6 January 2014. ISBN: 0393347818

To do or not to do

The first question might be "am I going to do anything?" Some people, for example, like to spend their time doing nothing. This is more common in some situations than overs. Lying doing nothing is more common at the beach or a warm summer's day in the park.

However, many people with anxiety struggle to switch off their minds. We find that doing nothing leads us into the trap of our mind constantly going back to those anxious thoughts. For us, spending an hour playing video games may be far more beneficial.

Good places to do nothing

If you fall on the side of *doing nothing* with your relaxation time, popular places to do this are:

- At the beach
- In the park
- In the bath
- On the sofa
- In a hot tub

Some of these are more accessible than others, of course. I do not have a hot tub in my house (or a park, or a beach).

Hierarchy of engagement

In my book *Technical Anxiety*, I discuss the different activities you can do and how effective they are at distraction. It comes down to how much engagement they require. For example, video games require a high level of engagement because you are controlling the game. In contrast, films require a low level of engagement because you can ignore them and they just continue playing.

When picking an activity to relax with, you need to select one that matches your personality. Do you need a high level of engagement or a low level?

Below, I have listed various activities and the engagement that they require.

Activity	Engagement
Films (and TV)	Low. You can just ignore the film entirely and think about something else. Even if you completely ignore it, it will continue to play.
Audiobooks	Low. Same as films.

Facebook	Medium. Can be quite a passive experience. You can just scroll through news feeds without paying much attention. Some posts may be engaging.
Reading	Medium. You do need to do the reading. However, it is easy to skim and not take in anything. Ever got the end of a page and realised you have no idea what you just read?
Conversation	Medium. You can hold a conversation while thinking about other things.
Housework	Medium. It does require you to do something but typically leaves you with enough cognitive capacity to think about other things. Also, most people would not consider doing housework as a relaxation exercise.
Video games	High. You have to pay attention and concentrate on most games. When you are in the thick of it, it is easy to forget what is going on around you.
Sport	High. Combines physical and mental attention.

Scheduling time

Like any activity, the best way to ensure relaxation gets done is to schedule time for it. Like putting aside an hour for exercise, allocating a particular time for relaxation helps ensure you do not miss your *you* time.

What counts as relaxing?

Relaxing is about giving your mind some time off. Therefore, a wide variety of activities may count as relaxing. You may not typically associate housework with relaxing, for example. However, if you find it gives your mind a break, it can be.

Here are five ideas that you might not consider relaxing, but which you may find therapeutic:

1. Cleaning and tidying the house
2. Washing the car
3. Sorting through old papers, letters, etc
4. Organising your books or DVDs
5. Tidying up your computer files

Deep relaxation

This time, I am talking about sitting with your legs crossed. ***Deep relaxation*** covers a range of techniques, including:

- Meditation
- Deep breathing
- Progressive relaxation

Opinions on the topic are divided. There is some evidence to suggest they are effective. However, the studies are often limited and of poor quality244. Most of all, it is difficult to generalise across a range of techniques treating a range of conditions.

I have discussed some in further detail here.

Meditation

Meditation may or may not be helpful. A Cochrane review concluded there was insufficient evidence for the benefits of mediation, both for physical health245 and for anxiety246. In the latter, they concluded:

"The small number of studies included in this review do not permit any conclusions to be drawn on the effectiveness of meditation therapy for anxiety disorders. Transcendental meditation is comparable with other kinds of relaxation therapies in reducing anxiety, and Kundalini Yoga did not show significant effectiveness in treating obsessive-compulsive disorders compared with Relaxation/Meditation. Drop out rates appear to be high, and adverse effects of meditation have not been reported. More trials are needed."

In any case, mindfulness meditation is a better more health-based approach with solid evidence behind it247. Therefore, regardless of how you feel

---

244 US National Center for Complementary and Integrative Health. Relaxation Techniques for Health. 12 January 2017. https://nccih.nih.gov/health/stress/relaxation.htm

245 Hartley L, Mavrodaris A, Flowers N, Ernst E, Rees K. Transcendental meditation for the prevention of cardiovascular disease. Cochrane Collaboration. 1 December 2014.

246 Krisanaprakornkit T, Sriraj W, Piyavhatkul N, Laopaiboon M. Meditation therapy for anxiety disorders. Cochrane Collaboration. 25 January 2006.

247 Hoge EA, Bui E, Marques L, et al. Randomized Controlled Trial of Mindfulness Meditation for Generalized Anxiety Disorder: Effects on Anxiety and Stress Reactivity. The Journal of clinical psychiatry. 2013;74(8):786-792. doi:10.4088/JCP.12m08083.

about meditation, pursuing mindfulness meditation instead would be the best option.

Yoga

Yoga is a traditional Indian system that uses a combination physical postures, breathing techniques, meditation and relaxation. Research on its overall benefits has so far been inconclusive248. Similarly, research specifically for anxiety concluded that more research was needed249.

However, you may enjoy yoga. It's not harmful, so if you like it, go ahead.

Progressive relaxation

There is currently no clear evidence that progressive relaxation is effective250.

Tracking your relaxation

So far in this book, I have suggested you track your exercise, diet and sleep. Can you guess what I am going to suggest next? Yes, it is to track your relaxation time.

Here is why you should keep a log:

- So that you know how much time you spend relaxing. Anxiety is am memory disorder. It will lie to you and tell you that you spent more time than you did.
- So that you can see what works best. Rate each relaxation session on a scale of 1-10. How relaxed do you feel afterwards? If one activity scores better than another, you may want to consider spending more time on it.

---

248 Smith, K. B. and Pukall, C. F. (2009), An evidence-based review of yoga as a complementary intervention for patients with cancer. Psycho-Oncology, 18: 465–475. doi:10.1002/pon.1411

249 G Kirkwood, H Rampes, V Tuffrey, J Richardson, K Pilkington. Yoga for anxiety: a systematic review of the research evidence. Br J Sports Med 2005;39:884-891 doi:10.1136/bjsm.2005.018069.

250 Jorm AF, Morgan AJ, Hetrick SE. Relaxation for depression. Cochrane Collaboration. 8 October 2008. DOI: 10.1002/14651858.CD007142.pub2

These results will inform how you spend your time. For example, you may find that your records show you spend a considerable amount of time on Facebook but do not rate it as a particularly pleasurable activity.

Meanwhile, you find that you spend little time listening to music, but that you rate it as a highly pleasurable activity. The action step here is obvious: spend more time listening to music and less time on Facebook.

It is only when you have the data that these patterns become apparent.

How to track online time

One of the issues with tracking your relaxation time is that it is often unplanned. You might sit down for 20 minutes without any real plan to do so. Do you record this? Ideally, yes. However, many of us will forget.

This is a difficult problem to fix in the real world. However, when it comes to what websites we browse, there is a solution. Installing a browser plugin that tracks website time will show you a summary.

What browser extension you use will depend on what browser you are using. I have included some suggestions below, but have not personally tested them all, so use whatever you see fit.

- Chrome: Be Limitless, timeStats, Time Tracker
- Firefox: Mind the Time, RescueTime
- Safari: WasteNoTime

The reason I make this suggestion is that I suspect most us feel we waste too much of our relaxation time online. Websites such as Facebook, Twitter, social media and newspapers (and guys, let's face it, pornography) probably consume more of our time than we would like. Seeing the cold hard numbers makes it easier to make different choices.

Remember that Facebook is in the business of delivering your eyeballs to advertisers. They try everything to keep you on their website. It is designed to be addictive.

Mindfulness in relaxation

Mindfulness can take two different forms when relaxing. The first is classic mindfulness meditation. I will not cover that in detail here but see my book *Technical Anxiety* if you want more information on how to do it.

The second is to ensure you are living in the present when undertaking relaxing activities. Remind yourself to focus on the task at hand, and the experiences and sensations it offers.

When I am relaxing, I often find myself thinking one of two things:

- I am not enjoying this. Therefore, I am going to brood on what a waste of relaxation time this is.
- I am enjoying this. Therefore, I am going to start counting down until this enjoyment is over.

When we find ourselves slipping into these thought patterns, we need to gently bring ourselves back to the present moment. There is no need to push the thought out: just let it slide on by and re-focus on what are you doing. I like to thank my mind and have a little chuckle about how silly it is.

It takes practice

There is an important lesson to take from these troublesome thoughts: relaxing takes practice. As I discussed in one of the previous sections, it does not come naturally to all of us.

It is very easy for our anxious minds to start worrying, even when we are doing something we enjoy. Letting these thoughts go and allowing them to pass before returning to the present moment takes time.

So, if you find that these thoughts are ruining all of your enjoyment, stay focused on the mindful techniques. Slowly but surely, you should see an improvement.

Such improvements will typically come in fits and starts. Some days you will feel better, and other days worse. But, the overall trend, should be positive. Tracking and rating your enjoyment should help you see a measurable difference, even if it does not always feel that way.

Summary

In this chapter, we reminded ourselves that relaxation is an enjoyable thing to do, and learnt that it has real, measurable health benefits.

It does not have to be some cross-legged meditation: any enjoyable activity that gives our mind a break will do. For best results, we should schedule relaxation time in and record how much we do and how effective it is.

While we are doing it, we need to remind ourselves to live mindfully and enjoy the moment.

Action steps

- Officially give yourself permission to relax.
- Schedule in regular relaxation time.
- Monitor how much time you spend and how effective it is. Do it for 30 days, then look at the results.

Personal growth

At one point or another, we all leave formal education. It is easy to think that this is the end of our learning. It is not. It is just the beginning. When we leave school it is the end of people telling us what to learn: but it is the start of life-long learning.

After this point, we can learn whatever we want. We are no longer constrained by a focus on the subjects that others think are important. We can pick what the topics about which we are passionate.

The downside: nobody is going to force us to do it. Often, they are not even going to give us the time. But it is critically important that we do do it. Learning new skills has a significant and positive impact on mental health[251].

Why is personal growth important?

The benefits of personal growth and lifelong learning include:

- Better health[252]
- Increased sense of purpose[253]
- Higher levels of social engagement[254]
- Improved ability to handle crises[255]

---

251 Mental Health Today, "The impact of adult and community learning programmes on mental health and wellbeing", https://is.gd/XOkklI

252 John Field. Is lifelong learning making a difference?Research-based evidence on the impact of adult learning. Second International Handbook of Lifelong Learning. Springer, Dordrecht, 2012. Pages 887-897.

253 Petra Herre. Benefits of Lifelong Learning (BeLL) study complete. European Lifelong Learning Magazine. 10 April 2014. http://www.infonet-ae.eu/articles-science-55/2150-benefits-of-lifelong-learning-bell-study-complete

254 John Field. Is lifelong learning making a difference?Research-based evidence on the impact of adult learning. Second International Handbook of Lifelong Learning. Springer, Dordrecht, 2012. Pages 887-897.

255 John Field. Is lifelong learning making a difference?Research-based evidence on the impact of adult learning. Second International Handbook of Lifelong Learning. Springer, Dordrecht, 2012. Pages 887-897.

- Greater probability of being in work256
- It makes you smarter257

Why is it beneficial for anxiety?

Personal growth provides a range of direct and indirect benefits258. Learning new skills is enjoyable, gives you a sense of achievement, builds confidence and strengthens social networks.

Research by the Mental Health Foundation suggested that adult learning had a positive impact for people with anxiety and depression due to promoting social relationships, building self-esteem and teaching people self-management strategies259.

Research by the London School of Economics suggested that education had a positive effect on mental health and that this was true regardless of age260.

Benefits for the long-term

One of the best findings of the research I mentioned in the introduction to this chapter, is just how long the benefits last.

Learning new skills does not just provide your mental health with a boost while you are learning. It lasts for years. You can still be gaining benefit from it a decade after you have taken a course.

---

256 Andrew Jenkins, Anna Vignoles, Alison Wolf and Fernando Galindo-Rueda. The Determinants and Effects of Lifelong Learning. April 2012. http://cee.lse.ac.uk/ceedps/ceedp19.pdf

257 The Royal Society. Neuroscience: implications for education and lifelong learning. February 2011.

258 John Field. Adult learning and mental well-being. Centre for Research in Lifelong Learning. University of Stirling.

259 Mental Health Foundation. Learning for Life: Adult learning, mental health and wellbeing. 2011. ISBN: 978-1-906162-66-5

260 Chevalier, Arnaud and Feinstein, Leon (2006) Sheepskin or prozac: the causal effect of education on mental health. CEEDP, 71. Centre for the Economics of Education, London School of Economics and Political Science, London, UK. ISBN 0753020181

What should I learn?

As I said in the introduction, once you leave school, nobody is scheduling your learning for you. This means that you are in full control. What do you **want** to learn? What will **you** find fulfilling? Below, I have included some suggestions.

Learn an instrument

I play guitar in a band called **The Assembly Line**. I am certainly not the ghost of Jimi Hendrix. However, I can hold a rhythm down, and occasionally bust out a bit of lead guitar as well261.

Here is the secret: I did not start learning to play the guitar until I was 27 years old. Playing guitar was not something I was naturally gifted at, nor had I learnt as a child. I ground it out. Within a year, I was playing with my band. Six months after that, I stopped my guitar lessons and picked up piano. Now I play the piano as well. Equally poorly, but I play.

There is no upper age limit on learning an instrument. In fact, research shows that people will into their retirement can pick up an instrument262.

What is the lesson here? That it does not matter if you are an adult. It does not matter if you have no musical aptitude. I was rubbish: I could not play a single song on the guitar for six months. But perseverance pays off. Natural talent is not a requirement.

Learn to cook

See the chapter on diet. Cooking is wonderful. It is my mindfulness. I love to lose myself in a recipe.

Learn a language

Languages are a very popular option. However, I am rather down on language learning. I have tried to learn to speak Finnish for years, and not made much progress. Nor is it as financially beneficial as people think263.

---

261 Chris Worfolk. The Assembly Line, November 2015. Chris Worfolk's Blog. 6 December 2015. http://blog.chrisworfolk.com/2015/12/06/the-assembly-line-november-2015/

262 David L. Crawford. The Role of Aging in Adult Learning: Implications for Instructors in Higher Education. New Horizons for Learning. December 2004. http://education.jhu.edu/PD/newhorizons/lifelonglearning/higher-education/implications/

However, one of the positive aspects of learning a language is that you typically do it in a group setting, and it gets you talking to lots of different people. Those are both highly beneficial.

Learn a new skill

Sometimes learning can be for both fun and profit. At the end of 2016, I realised I had a problem. I had just developed a course for people looking to become an IT contractor. I knew it was valuable because the people who went through the beta programme gave me positive feedback.

The problem was that nobody was using it because nobody knew about it. I knew that I could teach the material well, but I did not have the skills to promote it. So, I decided to learn marketing. It was a way to both help me sell my course **and** engage in some life-long learning.

The result? So far I love it. Not only am I learning, but I am learning with a purpose.

Learn to juggle

Juggling is an odd suggestion, I realise. However, it is a relatively easy skill to acquire. You can pick up the basics in a few hours of sustained practice: 30 minutes per day for a week. Watch "Learn How to Juggle 3 Balls" on YouTube264.

Learn a new sport

Personal growth does not have to involve academic learning. You could learn a new sport, or improve on an existing one.

Ways to learn

One feature that every plan needs is some actionable steps. How do we take action on personal growth? We look at some of the ways that we can learn.

---

263 Chris Worfolk. Is learning a foreign language really worth it? Chris Worfolk's Blog. 26 July 2016. http://blog.chrisworfolk.com/2016/07/26/is-learning-a-foreign-language-really-worth-it/

264 Learn How to Juggle 3 Balls. YouTube. https://www.youtube.com/watch?v=T16_BVIFFPQ

Books

A simple and classic method. If you want to learn about a topic, get a book on it. It is a cheap way to learn. You can typically buy a book for around £10, or you can visit your local library and get one for free.

Advantages:

- Low-cost
- Work at your pace
- There are lots of books on almost every topic

Disadvantages:

- Books are not always very engaging
- You have to provide all of the motivation
- There is nobody to help if you do not understand something

Online resources

Think books, but on the internet. They are often available for free and, again, are plentiful.

Advantages:

- Often free
- Some are a bit more interactive than books

Disadvantages:

- All of the same disadvantages as books
- It is hard to determine the quality of the resources

I will discuss some of my favourite online resources later in this chapter.

Private tutoring

If you want to put yourself on the fast track to learning and have the money to pay for it, private tutoring is a great option. I have used private tutoring to learning guitar, piano and Finnish.

Advantages:

- One-to-one support with an expert
- Can be at a time that suits you, and at your home
- Customised learning plan developed for you specifically

- You can ask questions and see demonstrations
- Tutor provides motivation to do your practice

Disadvantages:

- Expensive - typically £25+ per hour

Courses

Doing an "actual course" makes things seem a lot more real. This feeling makes it easier to do the work because there is a process to follow, a timeline to do it in and some oversight that you are doing the work.

There are lots of options here. It could be something fun. Something that leads to a qualification. Something that does both. Creative courses are consistently touted for mental health, but that is more important is that you do something in which you are interested.

Local community centres will run courses. These are often aimed at the retired or unemployed, and are, therefore, priced relatively cheaply. Mental health charities may also run courses specifically for people struggling with depression and anxiety.

Advantages:

- It feels more official because you go somewhere and do something
- It provides structure and routine
- You will often be learning in a group and making friends
- Less motivation required because the course instructor will have oversight
- The instructor is usually an expert who will be able to answer your questions
- May come with a certificate or qualification at the end

Disadvantages:

- Could cost money
- Less flexible learning
- Course start dates may be fixed to particular times of the year
- You may have to travel to a location
- You can only do the courses that are available in your area

University

Jack it all in and go back to university. Why not? Lots of people do. If you are happy with your current situation, it does not make sense to do this. However, if you feel you need to make a big chance in your life, this could be an option.

Advantages:

- Get to study something you are interested in for 3-4 years
- Earn a valuable qualification at the end
- In the UK, you can now get student loan to cover a masters degree

Disadvantages:

- You might feel out of place if you are older than 21 and doing an undergraduate course
- Very expensive, depending on where you do it (you could do a degree in Finland for free, for example)

MOOCs

MOOC stands for Massive Open Online Course. These are web-based courses in which anyone can participate. Some highly prestigious institutions now publish their courses online including Princeton, Stanford and MIT. Many are free of charge, and some even provide university credit265.

Advantages:

- Can provide a university-level education at a fraction of the cost
- Accessible, you do not have to leave your house

Disadvantages:

- Not usually recognised as real qualification
- May not provide oversight, tutoring or community

---

265 Major UK universities to award degree course credit through MOOCs for the first time with FutureLearn "Programs". 27 May 2016. http://www.open.ac.uk/republic-of-ireland/news/major-uk-universities-award-degree-course-credit-through-moocs-first-time-futurelearn-%E2%80%9Cprograms

How to learn

There are far better books than this on how to learn effectively. However, there are a few core ideas we should keep in mind that are important, but perhaps easy to forget. Therefore, I will remind us of them here.

Deliberate practice

K. Anders Ericsson, the man whose research forms the basis of the "10,000 hours rule", emphasises the importance of deliberate practice[266].

This means that if we want to improve a skill, we need to focus on improving it. This sounds obvious, but it is easy to miss the subtle difference.

I like to bake bread. However, for the majority of the loaves I bake, I am not improving my bread-making abilities. I am just doing the same thing I always do. This is also true for playing guitar, driving or photography. There is no focus for my activity; I am just going through the steps.

If I want to improve, I need to practice something a little more challenging deliberately. I need to push myself, take the time to review the results, and be willing to repeat the process until I have it correct. Once I have it down, I then need to repeat it until the new, improved way of doing this is just *the way* that I do it. This is how we learn and grow.

Case study

Jack wanted to improve his guitar skills. However, he also really enjoyed just having fun on the guitar. So he divided his schedule into two types of sessions.

There were practice sessions in which he would select a new skill, do exercises to develop that part of his playing, and repeat those exercises over and over again.

Then there were jamming sessions, in which he would play his favourite tunes. In these, he knew he was not doing much to improve, but was having more fun. Balancing out the two allowed him to develop his skills while staying motivated.

---

266 K. Anders Ericsson, Ralf Th. Krampe, and Clemens Tesch-Romer. The Role of Deliberate Practice in the Acquisition of Expert Performance. Psychological Review. 1993, Vol. 100. No. 3, 363-406.

Step-by-step

When trying to acquire new skills, it is important to break them down into individual parts that you can work on separately. Recall the earlier chapter when I discussed how my tutor teaches me piano. First, we do the hands individually, then we put them together, then we look at the tempo.

Your brain can only focus on one thing. Therefore, you need to break everything down to the level of *one thing* and practice that until you can do it without thinking about it.

This goes for academic learning, too. You need to learn about one concept, and then reinforce that concept until it is fully embedded inside your brain.

American football training

When I play American football, I sometimes play receiver. On the surface, it does not sound that complex. You run a preset route and catch the ball if thrown to you.

Digging deeper, there is far more to it. You have to set your feet up correctly, wait for the snap (the ball going into play), look at the right place, run the route, turn quickly and get your hands up in the correct shape to catch the ball.

Trying to learn all of these skills at once is impossible. The only way I can learn is to take them one at a time. We do drills for footwork, drills for turning, drills for getting out hands in the right position. Then we repeat them over and over again until we can do them without thinking. Only then can we bring them all together.

Learning is hard

I have already talked about my journey learning guitar. It was tough. I was rubbish at first. I practised for two hours per day, and even then it took me six months until I could play a simple song.

Then it all came together. Another six months after that and I was playing in a band. There were times in those first six months that I wanted to give up. Those feelings never go away completely. Even now, it is hard to pick up new stuff compared to playing the songs I know.

We all feel frustration and resistance when learning something new. The only way we learn is to remind ourselves of the end-goal and that everyone feels frustration. What we are going through is normal.

I will let you in on another secret: it is not supposed to be easy. Real, true value is created by hard work. If it easy to do this stuff, nobody would have anxiety. Or any other problems. We would all just float around with our head in the clouds, being amazing at everything.

This stuff is hard, and if you want to make a change, you have to step up and be willing to pay the price of hard work. All I can offer is a promise that it is worth it.

More ways to grow

So far in this chapter, I have talked a lot about learning. However, there are more ways to grow than gaining more knowledge in an academic context.

Anything that improves your knowledge, self-awareness, quality of life, fulfils aspirations or improves your social interactions could be considered personal growth.

That means that many of the other chapters in this book are also part of personal growth. Learning to look after your body through diet and exercise, or strengthening social relations, are all examples of personal growth.

So, if academic learning is not your forte, here are some other avenues you may wish to explore.

Sport & fitness

I have already discussed learning a new sport, and the idea of doing more physical activity in the exercise chapter. I am repeating the message again because it is an important one: sport, especially team sport, allows you to learn new skills, meet new people and improve your physical fitness.

Hobbies

Are there any hobbies or activities you enjoy, that you could become more invested in? It is easy to continue to do a hobby without getting any better at it.

Take photography, for example. I like photography and take a lot of photos. However, most of the time, I am not getting any better at photography. I am just taking the photos and not learning anything.

If I want to grow as a photographer, I need to focus. I need to pick a skill: maybe it is framing the photograph, using light or getting the most out of my filters. Then practice that skill until the knowledge is automatic.

Some people find this approach removes some of the fun. This is important because hobbies are supposed to be fun. Therefore, I find it best do a bit of both. Sometimes, I feel like developing my skills. At other times, I just want to mess around. They both have their place in my schedule.

Emotionally

This is such a big topic that I will deal with it in it a separate section.

Work

If you are in work, where do you want your career to go? You can ask this question at any level. I used to work at McDonald's. You can still have a plan. For some, their plan was to become a restaurant manager. For me, my plan was to work somewhere other than McDonald's.

There should be an overall goal, and steps for how to get there. For example, let's say that I decided I did want to become a restaurant manager at McDonald's. Here is how I could grow in my job:

- Volunteer to work on a wider variety of stations to improve my experience
- Use my knowledge to mentor and support newer colleagues
- Set progressive targets of being a floor manager, shift manager, assistant manager and finally restaurant manager

Those are ways to grow even if you are flipping burgers. If you have a salaried job, what is your plan and how can you achieve it?

If you are not in work, do you want to change that? If so, what steps could you take? What skills could you develop that would help you get back into work?

Leadership

In the chapter on community, I will discuss how you can gain enormous personal benefits by taking up a committee or leadership position within organisations.

Emotional growth

There are many different aspects of emotional growth. I will cover some of the key ones here.

Rationality

The ability to make rational decisions is a surprisingly tough one. As anxiety sufferers, we already know this, right? If we have a phobia, the chances are that we know it is an irrational fear, but we struggle to do anything about it.

One of the reasons for this is that the belief is formed by a combination of biological, social and emotional reasons, and the rational argument only comes later. In *The Believing Brain*267, author Michael Shermer argues that this is how we make **all** our decisions, not just the obviously irrational ones.

By default, we make emotional decisions. It takes a lot of effort to listen to the little voice inside our head that is talking about facts.

To illustrate, I will tell you a little story about my stand mixer. For clarity, a stand mixer is a kitchen appliance that you use for mixing cakes, kneading dough, whipping cream and a variety of other tasks.

I had two options. Option one was a KitchenAid mixer. It cost £800 and looked awesome. You could buy it in a variety of colours including raspberry, green apple, blue willow and ice blue. Oh, how beautiful they were.

Option two was a Kenwood mixer. It cost less, it had more features, and it has better product reviews. However, it was far less pretty than the KitchenAid mixer. I struggled with the question. I even wrote about it on my blog268. Which one to pick?

In the end, I decided to get the Kenwood. I made the correct decision, but it took months. This sounds like a stupid story, right? Well, in many ways, it is. However, there is some important stuff in here, too.

First, it was very hard to make the right decision. We should not underestimate that. Going with your head when your heart is pulling you in a different direction is difficult.

267 Michael Shermer. The Believing Brain: From Ghosts and Gods to Politics and Conspiracies How We Construct Beliefs and Reinforce Them as Truths. 24 May 2011. ISBN: 0805091254.

268 Chris Worfolk. Kenwood Chef KMC010. Chris Worfolk's Blog. 26 February 2016. http://blog.chrisworfolk.com/2016/02/26/kenwood-chef-kmc010/

Second, I was only buying a stand mixer. Imagine how much harder this would be with a major life decision in which I was far more **emotionally** invested. The effect scales up. The more it means something to you, the more difficult it is to make the rational decision.

So yes, a silly little kitchen appliance helped me grow emotionally. It was a little victory. But enough little victories add up. What little victories can you claim that will help you grow?

Setting and achieving goals

I have already talked about the importance of setting goals. However, it is worth considering exactly why setting and achieving those goals is good for our personal growth.

How well therapy works is affected by expectations. If you think a course of therapy will work, it is far more likely to be effective than if you do not269. Goals work the same way270.

Therefore, if we want to achieve our goals, in therapy or in life in general, we need to believe they are going to work. How do we gain this belief? Demonstrated proof.

In cognitive behavioural therapy, we demonstrate to ourselves that our anxiety is irrational by putting ourselves in uncomfortable situations and showing ourselves that it is not that bad. Over time, the lower levels of our brain finally get the message that the higher levels of our brain have been telling them for years.

We can apply the same technique here. Use graded exposure. Set yourself goals and follow through on them. If you fail to reach a particular goal, break it down into steps that you can manage. Repeat the process, hits lots of easy goals and build up to bigger goals.

---

269 Price M, Anderson PL. Outcome Expectancy as a Predictor of Treatment Response in Cognitive Behavioral Therapy for Public Speaking Fears Within Social Anxiety Disorder. Psychotherapy (Chicago, Ill). 2012;49(2):173-179. doi:10.1037/a0024734.

270 Jacquelynne S. Eccles and Allan Wigfield. Motivational Beliefs, Values, and Goals. Annual Review of Psychology. Vol.53:1-634 (Volume publication date February 2002). DOI: 10.1146/annurev.psych.53.100901.135153

Consistently hitting goals will teach your brain that you are someone who achieves their goals. That is a powerful mindset to take into any future opportunity.

Relationships

Growing in your relationships is a vital topic and one that I will be discussing in the chapter on relationships.

Openness

The ability to be honest with others, and allow them to be honest with you, is a hard fought battle. There is a reason that people are reluctant to give you their honest opinion: others usually react badly when they do.

I say that I would rather have feedback for improvement rather than compliments. Living that in practice, however, is hard. Emotionally, my ego craves the pat on the back, even though my brain knows that I would be much better served by asking for where I went wrong and how I can improve.

Developing this level of openness, and not getting caught up in feedback emotionally, is a muscle that takes time to build. It takes practice. It takes a gentle reminder every time we hear something we do not like.

Set yourself a challenge

In the chapter on exercise, I spoke about the idea of setting yourself a goal. This can be a powerful motivational tool. However, it can also become a distraction from your real goal of reducing your anxiety by changing your lifestyle.

The same thing applies here.

It can be useful to set yourself a goal so that you have something to work towards. For example:

- "I want to learn to play the drums so I can play in a local band with my friends."
- "I want to learn to speak some French so that I can take a trip to Paris and try it out."
- "I want to complete this course so that I can apply for a better job."

All of these provide you with motivation to continue growing when it gets tough (and it almost certainly will get tough, at some point or another).

However, as we discussed, it is a double-edged sword. If you find that the goal is getting in the way of doing what you want to do, it may be time to revise it.

Let's take the drumming example. Maybe you set out to play in a band, so you want to learn to read music at the same time. However, you find it so difficult that you struggle to find the motivation to practice because it is too stressful to practice the mechanics of drumming and reading music. In this case, it is time for a pivot: change your goal to being able to play without reading music. You can always reassess your goals at a later date. Goals are there to be helpful, not unhelpful.

Start small, and work up

Learning an instrument requires you to practice every day. That is a lot of practice. Think of the process as graded exposure: if you are not doing much learning at the moment, start small and work up. Learn to bake. You can drop in and out of that. Then build up to something bigger.

Five reasonably-quick skills to learn

1. Solving a 4x4 slider puzzle
2. Juggling with three balls
3. Tying a butcher's knot
4. Making honeycomb
5. Selling "hello" in five different languages

Objections to life-long learning

Most of us can come up with plenty of reasons why we do not want to engage in life-long learning:

- We don't want to have to find the space in our timetable
- We don't want homework
- We don't want the expense
- We don't want to do the research to find a course we want to do
- We don't want to face the possibility that we will pour time into something, not learn it, fail, and feel like we have wasted all of that time

I say reasons; I mean excuses. We all have ***excuses*** as to why we do not engage in life-long learning. But, now you know that your mental health depends on it, it might be time to push it up the priority list a little.

We all have the same 24 hours in a day. We have time for the things we **make** time for. Maybe the first step is scheduling in an afternoon to look at some courses. Then schedule in an evening to pick a course.

As for wasting time, note that the research says that doing the learning correlates with benefits. Not successfully completing the learning: just doing it.

Let's say you did fail. I have been trying to learn to speak Finnish for years. However, when my daughter was born, I gave up my lessons because I wanted to concentrate on my family. I had failed. Or had I? Even though I do not speak fluent Finnish, here are some benefits I gained from the experience:

- I speak a little bit of Finnish
- I made some new friends at Finnish Saturday school
- I endeared myself to my in-laws

Not to mention that the act of learning was beneficial to my mental health.

Online learning resources

I have already discussed some of the ways you can learn online. In this section, I wanted to mention some of my favourite places to visit on the internet.

Wikipedia

I love **Wikipedia** as a concept. Encyclopaedias used to be something only the rich could afford. Then, in 2001, Jimmy Wales and Larry Sanger came along and said: "let's take all human knowledge and make it available for free." Now the poorest people in the world have access to everything we know as long as they can get access to a computer or internet-enabled device.

It is a fountain of knowledge on almost any topic. Best of all, it gives you the chance to give back. If you can improve or add to an article, just hit the edit button and you can contribute your knowledge to the project.

YouTube

Video-sharing site **YouTube** has long been associated with endless cat videos. It is true that there are a lot of cat videos on there. However, there is a huge amount of learning resources on there as well.

When I was learning to play the guitar, I supplemented my in-person lessons with video tutorials from Justin Sandercoe and Marty Schwartz. When I am struggling with a cooking technique, I go to **YouTube** to see it in action. I even learned to fish using a YouTube tutorial.

Udemy

Udemy is an online learning platform to allows anyone to create a course. There are tens of thousands of them available, some free and some paid. I have used both and so far they have consistently been high quality and informative.

Coursera

Coursera have been successful in attracting several top universities to publish courses with them. Many of these courses are available for free, with the option to upgrade if you would like to receive a certificate.

Mindfulness in personal growth

Learning is an excellent chance to practice mindfulness.

Many of us find that concentrating on a topic that are not familiar with is a high resistance task. Therefore, it is common to find our minds wandering off, or negative thoughts about our ability to learn creeping in.

When this happens, remind yourself that it is natural for minds to wander, especially when they do not want to focus on the task at hand. Then gently guide your attention back to your learning and begin again.

The chances are that this will happen a lot. That is okay. Mindfulness is not about preventing your mind from wandering. It is about training it that you will return to the present moment. So, if you find yourself being constantly distracted, do not worry. Simply guide your mind back to the task and continue each time it happens.

Summary

In this chapter, we learnt that committing to a philosophy of personal growth and lifelong learning can help us stay physically and mentally healthy. These benefits are significant and long lasting.

We reminded ourselves that once we have left school, it is up to us to set our own curriculum. This means we can pursue things that excite us, but also puts the onus on us to be proactive.

Action points

- Brainstorm five ideas for courses or growth opportunities
- Set an end goal you want to work towards
- Pick your favourite idea and make a start

Relationships

If I could select the key ingredient of a healthy mind and body, it would be relationships. Not exercise, not diet, not any of the other factors in this book. Relationships are king.

It is easy to underestimate how important strong relationships are in your life. They add years to it. Whether someone is anxious or not, having strong relationships is one of the keys to health, longevity and happiness.

Why relationships are important

Relationships provide the same benefits that diet, exercise and other lifestyle factors do. Spending time with people you love is like spending time at the gym.

Relationships affect your life expectancy

Having strong relationships means you will live longer. Why this is the case is not clear. It could be that it is due, in part, to the psychological safety of having people to care for you[271]. Also, face-to-face contact causes the body to release oxytocin. I will discuss the benefits of this shortly.

Relationships affect your physical health

Strong relationships correlate with better overall health. Several different studies have shown specific benefits including lower blood pressure, lower risk of cancer, faster recovery from cancer and reduction of heart disease[272].

---

271 Ross CE, Mirowsky J. Family relationships, social support and subjective life expectancy. J Health Soc Behav. 2002 Dec;43(4):469-89.

272 Debra Umberson and Jennifer Karas Montez. Social Relationships and Health: A Flashpoint for Health Policy. J Health Soc Behav. 2010; 51(Suppl): S54–S66. DOI: 10.1177/0022146510383501

Relationships affect your mental health

Strong relationships play a vital part in allowing us to maintain good mental health. A research paper by the Economic & Social Research Council273 concluded:

"Adults with no friends are the worst off psychologically. There are significant health cost implications from the impact of this social isolation."

Nor is there any substitute for friends and family: being in education or employment does not replicate having an active social circle outside of these environments.

What benefits do relationships bring?

As well as improvementing your overall health, here are some specific reasons why having strong relationships is a good thing:

- Connecting with other people can make you feel more "normal".
- They can provide you with emotional support.
- It gives you the chance to provide them with emotional support, which is also important for your health.
- They can be someone to talk problems through with, work out solutions and put things in perspective.
- It can be an enjoyable way to spend time.

How do relationships provide benefit?

When you spend time with some face-to-face, it causes the body to release oxytocin. This is the same hormone that your body releases when you have sex or give birth.

Oxytocin is brilliant. It makes you happier, healthier and less anxious274.

---

273 Mental health and social relationships. Economic & Social Research Council. May 2013. http://www.esrc.ac.uk/files/news-events-and-publications/evidence-briefings/mental-health-and-social-relationships/

274 Kirsch P, Esslinger C, Chen Q, Mier D, Lis S, Siddhanti S, Gruppe H, Mattay VS, Gallhofer B, Meyer-Lindenberg A. Oxytocin modulates neural circuitry for social cognition and fear in humans. J Neurosci. 2005 Dec 7;25(49):11489-93. DOI: 10.1523/JNEUROSCI.3984-05.2005

The irony of social anxiety

Relationships are brilliant. But have you noticed something? Many of us suffer from *social* anxiety. Relationships are one of the things we struggle with. This, as I will explain, is neither an accident nor a coincidence.

Why do we feel social anxiety?

There is a reason that relationships are hard: they are important. Think of it from an evolutionary point of view. Back when we were early humans, it was crucial to stick together.

Being excluded from the group meant death. It meant not being able to protect yourself from predators. It meant not being able to work together to take down a woolly mammoth. It meant having no one to turn to for food when times were hard.

Running out of friends was like running out of food, water or shelter. It was the end of you. Mother Nature understands this and gives us an inbuilt worry about relationships. We fear exclusion[275]. As with all anxiety, some of us are a bit jumpier than others.

Surely that should make it easier?

You might think that if you were *more* worried about relationships and being excluded than other people were, that would make maintaining relationships easier. But it does not. Here is why.

It is not that we are bad at relationships. It is that we *think* we are, and find them difficult. Many people with anxiety are better at relationships than most people, thanks to our improved empathy and understanding.

However, we feel more paranoid about them. Because we are more likely to fear exclusion, we jump at every comment, every action, every facial gesture. We read more into situations than a muggle would.

Second, we no longer live in a world where being excluded means death. We can survive quite happily as hermits, never talking to anyone. This means we have the option to build relationships or not.

---

275 Susan Pinker. The Village Effect: How Face-To-Face Contact Can Make Us Healthier and Happier. March 2015. ISBN: 1848878583

What is the result? You take a person who is anxious about being excluded, and you give them a choice to build relationships or not. It is no surprise what we choose: we opt never to let ourselves get hurt in the first place.

The problem is that by avoiding building relationships, consciously or unconsciously, we are hurting ourselves in the long term because we deny ourselves all of the benefits that a strong social circle brings.

What relationships do I need?

There is a quote by Jock Elliot[276], a world champion of public speaking, that I love so much that I tend to quote in all of my writing about relationships.

"If I joined Twitter or Facebook I could have hundreds of brand new friends just like that. But how many of them would roll out a bed at 3 o'clock in the morning and come to my aid if I needed them?"

I love Friend Face. I think it is a wonderful tool for connecting and reconnecting with friends all over the world. However, having 1,000 friends on social media is no substitute for real world relationships.

You do not get the same oxytocin release from virtual relationships that you do from face-to-face ones[277].

We see the importance of this in gender differences. Men tend to have larger, less intimate social circles while women have smaller, more intimate circles. The result? Across the board, women live longer than men[278]. Relationships are just one factor in this, but they are certainly an important one[279].

---

276 Just So Lucky. Jock Elliott. 2011 Public Speaking World Championships. https://www.youtube.com/watch?v=m0a_EcZyQts

277 Susan Pinker. The Village Effect: How Face-To-Face Contact Can Make Us Healthier and Happier. March 2015. ISBN: 1848878583

278 Rita Ostan, Daniela Monti, Paola Gueresi, Mauro Bussolotto, Claudio Franceschi and Giovannella Baggio. Gender, aging and longevity in humans: an update of an intriguing/neglected scenario paving the way to a gender-specific medicine. Clin Sci (Lond). 2016 Oct 1; 130(19): 1711–1725. DOI: 10.1042/CS20160004

279 Hessler RM, Jia S, Madsen R, Pazaki H. Gender, social networks and survival time: a 20-year study of the rural elderly. Arch Gerontol Geriatr. 1995 Nov-Dec;21(3):291-306.

What counts as a strong relationship?

As a rule of thumb, a strong relationship is defined as "you can discuss your intimate problems, hopes and thoughts"280.

Friends and family that are less close are still beneficial. However, the most significant advantages are found in people you consider that close.

How close is close?

A good rule of thumb: how many friends would you consider asking to be the maid of honour or best man at your wedding.

How many do I need?

As many as possible, but ideally at least three281.

How do I build stronger relationships?

As we have already learned, face-to-face contact causes the release of oxytocin. This does not happen when chatting to someone on Friend Face. Therefore, face-to-face contact is critical to building strong relationships.

There is no big secret here. It is spending time with people. The more you put in, the more you get out.

Spend time on them

Building strong relationships takes time. The more time you spend, the stronger they will be. The time you put into a relationship is not only enjoyable (okay, sometimes it is not enjoyable) but also an investment in strengthening your relationship.

Active management

I do not leave my social connections up to chance. I have all my friends on a spreadsheet. I felt weird about it at first. My guess is that some people reading this will think "that is weird: you're tracking all of your social connections?".

---

280 Chris Worfolk. Technical Anxiety: The complete guide to what is anxiety and what to do about it. ISBN: 978-1539424215

281 Susan Pinker. The Village Effect: How Face-To-Face Contact Can Make Us Healthier and Happier. March 2015. ISBN: 1848878583

It's true. It also gets results.

Most people are bad at planning their social lives. They do not message me and suggest we get together. Yet, when I suggest it, they are always willing to meet up. There are two reasons why this could be the case:

1. They do not like me but are too polite to say "no, I don't want to hang out with you."
2. They don't have a spreadsheet

It could be that everyone I know has acute anxiety about upsetting me and so agrees to meet up even though they do not want to. However, option two seems far more probable to me.

Building relationships does not happen by accident. It takes planning. It is so easy in the modern world to allow a month to go by without seeing anyone. Put some time into planning your social calendar and reap the rewards.

Habit

We have already discussed how important habit is in getting things done. If you can get into a routine, it is just easier to follow through on virtually everything. Starting something new is hard; continuing something old is easy.

How can you use the power of habit to build your relationships? What about regularly scheduled meet-ups? Here are some possibilities:

*   Arrange to go for dinner at a family member's once per week
*   Join a social group that meets on a regular basis
*   Sit down every Monday and pick a friend or family member to arrange to meet up with (or several)

Even annual events can use the power of habit. We have regular parties that people know they can turn up to and plan their diary around:

*   Super Bowl
*   Eurovision
*   Halloween
*   New Year's Eve
*   Galileo Day

We meet up at other times, of course. However, having these habits means that even when life gets busy, we do not forget about socialising altogether.

How do I build closer relationships?

How do you become closer to someone? Again, there is no magic secret here. It is about putting in the leg-work.

Active listening

Too often I find myself not listening when I am in a conversation. I have my mind on something else. Or, I am already planning the next thing I am going to say. Both of these provide distractions from what the other person is saying.

These distractions result in us missing an opportunity to learn about the other person, and to respond in an appropriate way.

How do we avoid this? By using active listening[282]. This is not some complicated technology we need to learn. It is simply the idea of fully concentrating on what the other person is saying, comprehending it and responding appropriately.

Active listening involves eye contact and looking at the other person's body language[283], as well as the words and tone of their voice.

Self-disclosure

Sharing personal information about yourself helps build trust and understanding. It also invites the other person to share some information with you. This exchange is an essential part to close relationships[284].

There is no rush to self-disclose. Indeed, it is almost certainly better not to tell someone all of your intimate secrets on your first meeting. It should be done progressively over time. Critically, when someone self-discloses to you, it is important to maintain this confidence and keep the information private.

282 Christopher C. Gearhart and Graham D. Bodie. Active-Empathic Listening as a General Social Skill: Evidence from Bivariate and Canonical Correlations. Communication Reports Vol. 24 , Iss. 2,2011. DOI: http://dx.doi.org/10.1080/08934215.2011.610731

283 Roberston, Kathryn. Active listening: more than just paying attention. Australian Family Physician; Melbourne34.12 (Dec 2005): 1053-5.

284 Nancy L. Collins and Lynn Carol Miller. Lynn Carol Miller. Psychological Bulletin 116(3):457-75. December 2014. DOI: 10.1037//0033-2909.116.3.457

Later in this chapter, I will discuss talking to friends and family about anxiety.

Shared experience

Non-biological relationships (friends, lovers) are ones that are built entirely from shared experience. Every marriage freely entered into is held together solely by the memories of these experiences. Shared experience can strengthen biological relationships too.

How to build new relationships

So far we have discussed how to nurture relationships and strengthen existing ones. But what if you want to find and build new ones?

Putting yourself in the best position

As anxiety sufferers, the idea of going up to people in a bar and instantly making new friends may not be a scenario we could imagine. However, the truth is that almost nobody makes friends this way.

The majority of friendships are made through:

- School, university
- Work
- Neighbours
- Social groups and clubs

These partly arise because you find people with a shared interest (same degree programme, job, interest) and partly because of proximity: you build shared experiences with the people you spend time with[285].

Friends-of-friends

If I were to be callous, I would say that sifting through lots of people to find the ones you like is tedious. Or, to put it a nicer way, no matter how hard you try, you are not going to get along with everyone.

Why not use a shortcut? You like your friends, and they are likely to like people similar to you. So, why not make friends with their friends?

---

285 Bornstein, R. F. (1989). Exposure and affect: Overview and meta-analysis of research, 1968-1987. Psychological Bulletin, 112, 265-289.

How to build relationships when you have none

If you have no relationships, which is not uncommon for people with social anxiety, the idea of building new relationships can seem like an impossible task.

In this case, we need to take a cognitive behavioural approach and use some exposure therapy. In graded exposure, we break the process down into manageable chunks.

For example, could you start by building relationships online? The internet allows us to participant in relative anonymity. Online groups, forums, chat rooms, IRC and other platforms allow us to meet new people without leaving the house.

Once friendships are established, online groups often evolve into real-world meetings.

Support groups are also a great place to start. In the chapter on community, I will take more about the benefits of joining a local anxiety support group.

Building relationships requires some discomfort. There is no way around it, unfortunately. However, we can keep that discomfort to manageable levels by breaking it down step-by-step.

Talking about anxiety

There are few things more therapeutic than being able to unload. That is the basis for talking therapy, after all. However, many people feel that they cannot talk to anyone about their anxiety, especially their friends and family. This situation is unfortunate because it is often the **best** thing you can do.

Talking to your family

There are two excellent reasons to talk to your family about it. One is that they probably love you very much.

If this is not true, well, that's a tough hand you have been dealt. No wonder you have anxiety. However, for most people, their family are the people who love them most of all. Therefore, if you are going to get compassion, understanding and support, this is the place to do it.

Second, the research shows that you can be genetically predisposed to anxiety286. When you go digging, you never know what you will find. It may be that you are not alone in your struggle with anxiety. I wasn't. Having a bonding experience like that brings you closer together.

Talking to your partner

If you are in a relationship, talking to your partner is critical. Expressing your emotions will build a stronger relationship while suppressing your emotions has been shown to have an adverse effect on your relationship287.

It is a hard conversation to have: but the future of your relationship may depend on it.

Talking to your children

As a parent, you may experience a natural feeling that you need to be strong for your children and keep your anxiety covered up. This feeling is entirely natural. Just like anxiety is natural. However, it is also, in my opinion, a bad idea.

Hiding anxiety from your children forces you to lead a double life. One in which you are the real you and the other in which you are a super-parent, not afraid of anything.

Being honest with them has some advantages:

- You relieve the psychological pressure of trying to keep it hidden.
- You do not have to explain any weird behaviour that pops up as a result of your anxiety.
- You expose your children to the idea that it is okay to talk about mental health.

---

286 Scherrer, Jeffrey F. et al. Evidence for genetic influences common and specific to symptoms of generalized anxiety and panic. Journal of Affective Disorders, Volume 57, Issue 1, 25 - 35. DOI: http://dx.doi.org/10.1016/

287 Todd B. Kashdan, Jeffrey R. Volkmann, William E. Breen, Susan Han. Social anxiety and romantic relationships: The costs and benefits of negative emotion expression are context-dependent. Journal of Anxiety Disorders 21 (2007) 475–492.

Talking to friends

Friends are people who choose to spend time with you. They are not socially obliged to: they do it because they want to. That means they are people who like you and enjoy your company.

Because of this, friends are an ideal candidate to open up to about your anxiety. You do not have to do it all at once. You could start with one friend that you think will be particularly supportive. They have already put up with your craziness so far, so are likely to stick with you through this.

Friends can be useful both for emotional support but also when doing activities such as exposure therapy. Let's say you have social anxiety and your therapist helps you break down your graded fear list. Before you "go to the party on your own and stay all night" you probably have "go to the party with a friend and stay for 30 minutes". You need a friend for that.

So, tell them about your anxiety and see what happens. They may have their own stories. They may simply be supportive. You never know until you try.

Helping people understand

Opinion is divided on how difficult it is to emphasise with anxiety. Some people think that if you have never experienced a panic attack, it is hard to imagine what it is like.

Other people point out that everyone has experienced some level of anxiety. If it does not interfere with your life, you may struggle to see what the big deal is. After all, you have *a bit* of anxiety, and it is fine.

Which view is correct? Maybe a mixture of both.

How do we help the people in our lives understand what we are going through?

One way, and this is the way I most recommend, is buying them a copy of my book *Technical Anxiety*288 and telling them to read the chapter for friends and family. However, I fully accept that I am extremely biased in this opinion.

---

288 Chris Worfolk. Technical Anxiety: The complete guide to what is anxiety and what to do about it. ISBN: 978-1539424215

Aside from that, here are some top tips:

- Acknowledge the fact that it is hard to understand. Too often I see people post memes on Facebook about how people should just understand how it feels. The truth is, I have no idea that **Chronic fatigue syndrome (ME)** feels like. You need to explain it to me, and still, I probably will not get it. Anxiety is like that too: it is not obvious to muggles.
- Talk through an anxiety-proving scenario. How do you feel? What symptoms do you experience? What hurts, and where does it hurt? Put it in terms of bodily sensations that others can imagine.
- Tell them how they can help, and what is not helpful. Do you want them to make supportive comments? Do you want them to just be there? Let them know so it is clear how they can be most supportive if they want to be.

Managing anxiety and relationships

I'll let you in on a big secret: you do not have to be a perfect friend all of the time. I bet people have not always been a perfect friend to you, right? But you are still friends with some of them? Friends understand.

It is okay to let someone down once in a while. If you wake up and find that you cannot face the world, then you cannot face the world. It is not your fault.

Here are some thoughts that may go through your head when you let someone down:

- I am a terrible friend
- I have let them down
- They will not like me anymore
- They will think I am a bad person
- I am embarrassed
- I do not think I can face them anymore

Believe it or not, there are **exactly** the thoughts that someone with anxiety would have. Understand that that is the reason you have them. Not because they are true (there may be a little truth in some of them, but nobody is perfect) but because that is the thought patterns that anxiety sufferers encounter.

Muggles, on the other hand, just do not worry about it that much. If you do let someone down, that just makes you an average person. It is just that you beat yourself up about it more than most.

Mindfulness in relationships

So far, in our discussions about mindfulness, we have focused on ourselves. It is about what our mind is doing and what we are thinking. With relationships, it is not all about you.

We want to use mindfulness to support others. When we are spending time with people, we want to live in the present moment to give them our full attention. When we are in conversation, we want to actively listen to what they are saying, and not just be a passive participant.

Gratitude

Another way we can employ mindfulness to improve our relationships is by cultivating gratitude. This means reminding ourselves how thankful we are for the existing relationships in our lives. These relationships could be your family, partner, friends or anyone else that you are grateful for being in your life.

Developing feelings of gratitude leads to better mental health[289] and improved mood[290].

You can help develop gratitude by:

* Thinking about gratitude in mindfulness meditations[291]
* Telling people you are grateful for their friendship, or writing them letters[292]

---

289 C. Nathan DeWall, Nathaniel M. Lambert, Richard S. Pond, Todd B. Kashdan, Frank D. Fincham. A Grateful Heart is a Nonviolent Heart. Social Psychological and Personality Science. Vol 3, Issue 2, 2012.

290 Robert A. Emmons, Michael E. McCullough. Counting Blessings Versus Burdens: An Experimental Investigation of Gratitude and Subjective Well-Being in Daily Life. Journal of Personality and Social Psychology. 2003, Vol. 84, No. 2, 377–389. DOI: 10.1037/0022-3514.84.2.377

291 Mark Williams, Danny Penman. Mindfulness: A Practical Guide to Finding Peace in a Frantic World. 5 May 2011. ISBN: 074995308X

292 Steven M. Toepfer, Kelly Cichy, Patti Peters. Letters of Gratitude: Further Evidence for Author Benefits. J Happiness Stud. DOI: DOI 10.1007/s10902-011-9257-7

- Keeping a journal, and noting down three things each day that you are grateful for293

Summary

In this chapter, we learnt that building strong relationships is probably the most important thing you can do for maintaining good mental health and a happy life.

We looked at why people with anxiety often struggle with relationships, and some of the ways we can work around that. Finally, we looked at talking about anxiety with others.

Action points
- Review how actively you are managing your relationships
- Start a new habit that will make regular social contact easier
- Use active listening to engage more with others
- Use a system to develop gratitude for the relationships you have
- If you are looking to make new friends, put yourself in the best possible position by spending time with other friends and joining social groups

---

293 Joshua A. Rash, M. Kyle Matsuba, Kenneth M. Prkachin. Gratitude and Well-Being: Who Benefits the Most from a Gratitude Intervention? Volume 3, Issue 3. November 2011. Pages 350–369. DOI: 10.1111/j.1758-0854.2011.01058.x

Community

Community is relationships on a wider scale. However, it is also more than that. Being part of a community brings together many of the benefits we have already discussed in this book: it provides routine, structure, social connections, a sense of purpose and a reason to get out of the house.

Being part of something bigger helps you take your mind away from introspection and towards a more fulfilling purpose of being part of something broader.

Why is community important?

We have already discussed the extensive benefits of building and maintaining relationships. Community is also a connector: it combines relationships, personal growth and going outside.

Being part of a community reminds you that you are part of something bigger. It is not all about you. Participating helps get you out of your own head, which makes you feel better[294]. It develops the social and psychological resources that prevent depression[295].

Contributing to a community builds your self-esteem[296] and make and makes you feel better[297]. In a 2003 survey, more than four in five people said they felt volunteering had a positive impact on their mental health[298].

---

294 Whitney L. Heppner, Michael H. Kernis, Chad E. Lakey, W. Keith Campbell, Brian M. Goldman, Patti J. Davis, Edward V. Cascio. Mindfulness as a means of reducing aggressive behavior: dispositional and situational evidence. Volume 34, Issue 5. September/October 2008. Pages 486–496. DOI: DOI: 10.1002/ab.20258

295 Marc A Musick, John Wilson. Volunteering and depression: the role of psychological and social resources in different age groups. Social Science & Medicine. Volume 56, Issue 2, January 2003, Pages 259–269. DOI: http://dx.doi.org/10.1016/S0277-9536(02)00025-4

296 Michal (Michelle) Mann, Clemens M. H. Hosman, Herman P. Schaalma, Nanne K. de Vries. Self-esteem in a broad-spectrum approach for mental health promotion. Health Education Research. Volume 19 Issue 4. August 2004. DOI: https://doi.org/10.1093/her/cyg041

297 Arnstein P, Vidal M, Wells-Federman C, Morgan B, Caudill M. From chronic pain patient to peer: benefits and risks of volunteering. Pain Manag Nurs. 2002 Sep;3(3):94-103.

Support groups

One of the best places to start is by joining a local support group, such as the charity I run, Anxiety Leeds. In this section, I will explore what exactly a support group is and how they tend to operate. However, each one is different, and you may even find a range of different groups in your local area.

Types of support groups

Peer support: In this setting, a group would be organised by a facilitator, but they would take no leadership role. There is no teaching: group members can share their experiences and offer each other advice.

Enhanced peer support: This is a bridge between peer support and group therapy. In this context, it would be member-led and overseen by a facilitator. However, the facilitator would typically be a professional or exceptionally knowledgeable individual who could provide authoritative advice.

Group therapy: In this setting, a group would meet for a fixed period, for example, every week for 12 weeks. The group would be lead by a professional, but there would usually be an emphasis on group members supporting each other.

Social group: These are groups that take place outside of any formal setting. They may meet in a pub, for example, but with an understanding that it was for people with social phobia or other anxieties and with an emphasis on supporting each other.

How Anxiety Leeds works

Our support group is pretty typical of the peer support format you may encounter at other groups. Therefore, I will describe it in some detail to give you an idea of what you can expect elsewhere.

We meet on a fortnightly basis at a local hospital. We have two facilitators, who get there a little earlier and set out a ring of chairs. We all sit facing each other so that everyone can see, get the chance to speak, and feel included.

298 Sherry Clark, (2003) "Voluntary work benefits mental health", A Life in the Day, Vol. 7 Iss: 1, pp.10 - 14. DOI: http://dx.doi.org/10.1108/13666282200300005

Everyone who attends the group is an anxiety sufferer, including the facilitators. We also allow people to bring a friend or family member along to support them. This means that if someone is too anxious to attend for the first time by themselves, they can come with a loved-one to get them in the door.

We do not allow health professionals, researchers, students or any other non-anxiety sufferers to attend the group. This policy ensures that everyone there can personally relate to the issues being discussed and provide empathy and support.

We run the group in a drop-in format. This means that people do not have to book in advance: they can just turn up on the night. This setup is pretty typical, though some groups may have more formal rules, especially when you attend for the first time.

We have used a number of different formats over the years. Historically, we have had no topic. People can turn up and discuss any issues affecting them. We have also tried having a meeting theme, such as "sleep" or "making positive changes". Other times, we divide the meeting into two: half for an open session and half for a theme. Even when there is a theme, other topics are not off limits: it is just a guide to something we may want to discuss.

Why join a support group?

Support groups offer some advantages above and beyond what you can gain from other social groups.

It gives you a place to talk. People with anxiety often feel like they cannot talk to their friends and family about it because they think they will get fed up of hearing about it. Whether this is the case (often it is just the anxiety talking), there is no fear of this at a support group: that is the whole point of the group existing.

You can access a higher level of empathy. Friends and family are likely to offer love and support. However, if they have not experienced anxiety themselves, they may not be able to appreciate exactly how it feels. At a support group, everyone else has been through it and knows exactly how you feel.

People can offer you advice and stories from their experience. About to start CBT and unsure what to expect? The chances are that someone at the group has already been through it and can tell you about it. Whether it is drugs, therapy, alternative remedies or any other experience, someone somewhere will have tried it and be able to report back.

You will feel relieved that it is not just you. You are not the only person going through this. Just listening to other people describing their experiences and discussing their symptoms can be therapeutic because you realise that they are going through the same things you are.

It puts your anxiety in context. It is easy to feel like anxiety is ruining your life. However, often, other people have it even worse. Or maybe you have managed to do something they have not. It is a gentle reminder to celebrate your achievements, even if they feel really tiny to you.

You pick up all kinds of useful information. Did you know that anxiety is classified as a long-term health condition, which falls under disability discrimination law in the UK? I did not. Not until someone at my support group told me.

It is a supportive place to go for people with social anxiety. It is a great alternative to going to the pub, or a party, or other high-anxiety situations where nobody will understand how you feel. Support groups are gentle by design and provide you with an understanding audience who will be supportive about the difficulties of dealing with social situations.

Tips for attending your first meeting

One of the problems with having anxiety is that going to a room full of strangers can be very anxiety provoking! Below, I have included a few tips for getting yourself through the door for the first time.

1. Conduct a trial run beforehand. If you are worrying about attending the meeting and worrying about how to find the room, that is a lot of things to stress about. Cut them in half by finding out where the room is in advance.
2. Arrive early, or late. Arriving early allows you to find the place and then calm down before you have to face the meeting. I use this technique for handling job interviews. If you are worried about awkwardly standing around before the meeting starts, you could also arrive late. Anxiety Leeds runs in a drop-in format, so you can turn up whenever you want.
3. Remember that you do not have to say anything. Most groups allow people simply to listen to other people's stories, and this in itself can be beneficial. You can always speak at a later meeting if you decide you want to.
4. Take someone with you to support group. Most groups allow you to bring a friend or family member along for emotional support.

5. Do not worry if you do not make it. Most people that contact us at Anxiety Leeds never turn up. Others come to the hospital, but it takes them a couple of meetings to get in the door. This is normal. Think of it like exposure therapy: each time you can go a little further.

Community groups

It is not just support groups that are beneficial for anxiety. Joining any group is useful and provides a host of benefits.

- It provides you with a reason to get out of the house
- It provides structure and routine
- It gets you interacting with other people and provides a chance to make new friends
- It provides opportunities for learning and personal growth
- It allows you to develop a good behaviour: set yourself a goal of attending and then follow through on that goal

Finding community groups

It used to be the case that if you were interested in joining a group, you would go down to your local library and look at the listings. Those days are long gone: now everything is available to find on the internet.

If you know what you are looking for, then search:

- Google
- Facebook

If you want to be inspired by new ideas, then browse:

- Meetup.com
- BBC Sport Get Inspired (UK-based)

Five suggestions

Here are five suggestions for groups you might want to consider.

Public speaking clubs: Nothing builds up confidence like a public speaking club. It is a big fear for many people, so the chance to overcome it can be incredibly empowering. Most speaking clubs are geared up for new and nervous speakers (don't start with the Professional Speakers Association, for example) and will provide the same kind of support you get at a peer support group.

Drama groups: These hit a lot of the key points for mental health. It allows you to be expressive, it is fun, and it helps build confidence.

Choir: Choirs are hip and modern these days. They sing pop songs. It helps you develop your voice and teaches you a new skill. You can be part of a group at first, and move on to doing solos if you are smashing it. You can push your boundaries with performances. Or, you can just turn up each week and have some fun.

Language groups: Want to learn a foreign language? There is no better practice than being able to use your skills on others, especially native speakers. Such groups are often open to both native speakers and those trying to learn, so make excellent places to refine your skills.

Reading groups and book clubs: These are useful because you can drop in and out as books take your interest, and always provide you with a topic of conversation (no awkward silences).

How to get the most out of community

A large part of involvement with community activities is *just turning up*. That in itself can be difficult for us, though. Many of us do not feel confident in social situations, so this can be tough.

It is going to be hard at first

Like taking medication, the benefits of community are unlikely to appear on day one, but the side effects will.

The first time you go to any new group, it is going to be anxiety provoking. You may not know anyone there. It takes time to build relationships and make new friends. These benefits will come later down the line. On day one, you will probably feel awkward and out-of-place.

Remind yourself that this is normal and that it is only by pushing through this that you will gain the benefits.

Commit to attending

Throughout this book, I have repeatedly emphasised the importance of habit and routine. If you decide to join a new group, make it part of this routine.

Commit to going on a regular basis. Doing this reduces the mental strain of *deciding* whether you want to go each time. It prevents the internal discussion of the benefits and drawbacks. Try it say half a dozen times, and then evaluate whether you are enjoying it or not.

Giving back

A core part of being in a community is not only taking from it, but also giving back. At first glance, this appears to be paying your dues for what you have received. But it is of benefit to you, too: giving back actually helps you as much as the people to which you give.

Taking a leadership role

Taking a leadership role in a group has even more benefits than attending them. These include:

- Building your confidence and self-esteem even further
- A chance to learn new skills
- Additional tasks to take your mind off your anxiety
- A positive feeling of giving back to the community

When you join a new group, you may think that the organisers are experts, or seasoned veterans, or appointed by a special council of elders. This may be true. Usually, though, they are just regular people who stepped up to the plate.

Therefore, you should not feel like you have to wait until you feel you know everything before getting involved. You have anxiety: the chances are that day will never come.

Let's say you join a group that has a committee, and that committee is elected once per year. Can you run for the committee if you only joined the group three months ago? Of course! I can tell you from personal experience that I would much rather have someone with enthusiasm and who wanted to get involved and help out than have someone with experience. It's a community group: turning up is half the battle.

Leading a peer support group

An excellent way to get involved in community leadership is to become a facilitator at your local peer support group. You are the perfect candidate for the job: someone with experience of anxiety that can help the meetings run smoothly.

Because we all have a background of anxiety, we know how frustrating and intense it can be. Having the chance to help others with that and make a real difference in people's lives is a powerful boost to your self-esteem.

I have found that running **Anxiety Leeds** has also been very helpful for my anxiety. Sharing my experiences, coping strategies and solutions helps reinforce the knowledge in my mind. Doing this makes it easier to execute these strategies in the real world.

The benefits of giving back

When we serve our community, we are rewarded with respect, influence and power.

People often think of power in the Machiavellian sense: people scheme and achieve it by force. However, Dacher Keltner argues this is incorrect. Power and influence are given as rewards when people act selflessly (and is taken away just as fast when they do not!).

When you act altruistically, people value you. They reward with you more respect and a higher standing in society. Ironically, the only way to achieve this is genuinely to act selflessly, without expecting a reward.

What is the result of this new-found respect? We live happier, healthier and longer lives299.

Ways to help others

Running groups is one way of giving back. However, there are lots of different ways. Here are ten suggestions:

1. Spend time with a friend or relative that could use some company. Even phoning them is helpful.
2. Cook a meal for the people you live with, or a friend.
3. Have a clear out and donate the items to a local charity shop.
4. Offer to babysit.
5. Do some dog-walking at your local animal shelter.
6. Pick up litter at your local park. You do not need permission.
7. If someone you know is nervous about an event, offer to go with them.

---

299 Dacher Keltner. The Power Paradox: How We Gain and Lose Influence. 17 May 2016. ISBN: 1594205248

8. Use your knowledge to provide answers to people on internet Q&A boards such as Quora, Yahoo Answers, Stack Overflow, etc.
9. Spend a morning volunteering as a marshall at Parkrun.
10. Take the time to thank someone who has done something nice for you recently.

Work

Many people with anxiety struggle to hold down a job. This is a shame because work provides a significant boost to your mental health300. Benefits include:

- A stable routine
- Regular social contact with colleagues and customers
- A reason to get up in a morning
- Gets you out of the house
- A sense of purpose and self-worth
- Keeps your mind occupied

Objections to community

Worried about increasing your participation in the community? I would be surprised if you *were not* a little apprehensive. Below, I have provided reasons why you should push through this feeling.

I will not enjoy it

It's true; you may not enjoy it at first. It takes time to feel like you know what is going on, and build the friendships that make community participation worth it. So, initially, it may not be that fun.

However, this will change over time. Also, regardless of fun, it starts being good for you from day one.

Attending x is anxiety-provoking

Again, this is probably true. However, this is not a reason *not* to do it. Quite the opposite. This is an excellent opportunity for us to grow as a person. It is a chance to challenge our anxiety.

---

300 Australasian Faculty of Occupational & Environmental Medicine. Realising the health benefits of work – An evidence update. November 2015.

If you feel this is too much, we need to go back to the idea of graded exposure. How can you break it down? Can you bring a friend to support you? Can you just attend part of the event? Is there a different activity with which you could start?

I do not have time

I discussed this in the chapter on relaxation. We all have the same 24 hours in the day. We have time for the things that we make time for. Do you *choose* to prioritise looking after your health, or is that not important to you?

There is one caveat to this. Some people with anxiety, use community to escape. They get involved in dozens of groups. I should know: I have done it. In this case, I would not encourage you to take on anything new, unless the groups you are already involved with are getting all of the attention and time that they deserve.

I am not good enough to lead

Come on; I am sure you can see the thinking error here. You might counter that by saying "but I really am not good enough: I have evidence for it". In this case, you are the *most* in need of taking on a leadership role. Why? Because it builds confidence and self-esteem.

As I discussed in the section on giving back, community groups need people who are willing to put in some time and enthusiasm. They do not need experts. They are not paying you to be a world-class professional. You are good enough, and even if you weren't, practise will make you into that person.

I do not want any responsibility

That is an understandable feeling. For anxiety sufferers, this is a sign you should take on some responsibility, though. Having to worry about other things gets us out of our head. I will discuss this more in the section on mindfulness.

Mindfulness and community

As anxiety sufferers, we spend a lot of time in our head. One of the key aspects of community, is to get us out of there. We need to remind ourselves that life is not all about us.

Community gives us the opportunity to contribute to something bigger and greater than ourselves. It takes our mind off our difficulties, and onto the bigger picture301.

When engaging in community activities, gently remind yourself that the world is much bigger than your head and that it feels good to be a part of something bigger.

It does not always feel good

I usually find community and volunteering opportunities a worthwhile activity to be a part of. But not always. Sometimes, a meeting of Anxiety Leeds rolls around, and I do not want to go out and spend my time there when I could just stay at home in bed.

At such times, I could remind myself that attending a support group is beneficial for me personally. However, a more effective tactic is to remind myself that it is not just about me: the people who attend the group are relying on the facilitators to be there to help them feel better.

This is not a stern "buck up and get over yourself." It is a gentle reminder that to be the good person I want to be, I need to consider the feelings of others. The fact that it *also* improves my health302 is an irrelevant, but welcome, bonus.

Cultivating an attitude of humility tends to make people happier and more successful303.

Summary

In this chapter, we learnt that community can provide for many of our needs, including social, personal growth and building self-esteem.

We reviewed the value of being part of a support group, the advantages of participating in community groups, and the benefits of taking a leadership role.

301 NHS Choices. Should I volunteer? 11 August 2015. http://www.nhs.uk/LiveWell/volunteering/Pages/Whyvolunteer.aspx

302 Terry Y Lum, Elizabeth Lightfoot. Effects of volunteering on the physical and mental health of older people. Research on Aging 27(1):31-55. January 2005. DOI: 10.1177/0164027504271349

303 Ryan Holiday. Ego is the Enemy. 14 June 2016. ISBN: 1591847818

Action points

- Join a local anxiety support group
- Join other local community groups
- Commit to attending on a regular basis
- Take a committee or leadership role in at least one of them

Conclusion

Let's re-cap what we have learnt in this book:

1. The best way to manage anxiety is through lifestyle.
2. We can measure our lifestyle on seven metrics: exercise, diet, sleep, relaxation, personal growth, relationships and community.
3. The way to improve these things is to pick one specific action, make the change until it becomes a habit, then rinse and repeat.
4. Doing this gradually builds up a compounding effect that allows us to live, happier, healthier, less anxious lives.

That's all there is to it. I would say "it's that simple", but that is misleading. There is no complex logic here. However, that would undermine how difficult it can be to make a change. This book is easy to read, but difficult to follow through on.

Whether you make these changes is up to you. I cannot do it for you. So, it is time to set your first goal: implement the things you have learnt from this book. Make it a goal. Write it down. Action it before you drop this book on the pile.

You did not learn to let anxiety rule your life overnight. It took a long time. Reversing this is a slow process, too. It is hard work and requires regular attention. We need to set those expectations at the start.

However, like graded exposure, we can break everything down into small, manageable steps. Over time, these changes add up until you achieve things you may not yet believe you are capable of.

The rest of your life is waiting. What do you choose?

About the author

Chris Worfolk is the founder of mental health charity **Anxiety Leeds**304. The organisation facilitates peer support groups for people struggling with anxiety and panic attacks.

In 2016, Chris founded **Worfolk Anxiety Management** and published **Technical Anxiety: The complete guide to what is anxiety and what to do about it**305. The book offers a comprehensive introduction to anxiety including what it is, how it works and what treatment is available and how to manage it.

He lives in Leeds, United Kingdom with his wife and daughter.

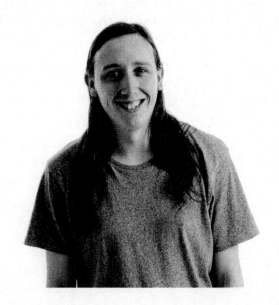

304 Anxiety Leeds. About Us. http://www.anxietyleeds.org.uk/about-us/

305 Chris Worfolk. Technical Anxiety: The complete guide to what is anxiety and what to do about it. ISBN: 978-1539424215

Glossary

Acute anxiety: Acute means severe or intense. In the case of acute anxiety, this means anxiety is that is considered severe enough to be a medical condition.

Amygdala: An area of the brain. It is part of the limbic system. It is responsible for decision making, memory and emotional reaction on a low level. This is different to higher-level reasoning, which is much more well informed. The amygdala makes simple, emotionally-driven decisions.

Benzodiazepines: A type of drug. *Benzos*, as they are also known, are a sedative. They are sometimes prescribed for anxiety. However, due to their short-term effects and being highly addictive, they should only be used for a few weeks at a time.

Causation: Cause and effect. Causation refers to one thing causing another. This is often confused with correlation. See *correlation* for a full definition.

CBT: See cognitive behavioural therapy.

CBT-I: Cognitive behavioural therapy for insomnia. This is a particular form of CBT developed for dealing with sleep problems.

Chronic: An illness that persists or consistently recurs.

Chronic fatigue syndrome (CFS): Also known as *myalgic encephalomyelitis (ME)*. A severe and long-term illness in which people find themselves feeling exhausted even after sleeping or resting.

Clinical anxiety: See *acute anxiety*.

Cognitive behavioural therapy (CBT): One of the most widely used therapies for anxiety and depression. CBT includes both looking at your thinking (the cognitive side) and your actions (the behavioural side).

Cognitive therapy: A form of therapy for anxiety and depression that looks at your thoughts. It was first developed in the 1960s. It has since been superseded by *cognitive behavioural therapy (CBT)* that includes the cognitive aspects.

Cohort study: A study that takes a set of people and follows them over time. For example, you could take a set of people who went to university and track them for 20 years to see if they earn more. If they do, this does not prove that university causes people to earn more because it could be other factors (we see correlation, not causation). However, it does suggest that they may be related. When we cannot do double blind trials, cohort studies are the next best alternative.

Control group: A group of participants in an experiment who receive no treatment or a fake treatment. See **placebo effect** for more details.

Correlation: Two things that occur together, but are not necessarily causative. For example, when umbrella sales go up, it is likely to rain. That does not mean that umbrella sales **cause** it to rain. However, if you just look at the data without wider context, it is easy to jump to that conclusion. In reality, we know it is the other way round. When two things correlate, one may cause the other, or they may be unrelated. Only a study to show **causation** can prove this.

Cortisol: A hormone, often known as the "stress hormone". Having too much cortisol in your system is bad for your health. Relaxation can reduce cortisol levels.

Dietary counselling: A kind of therapy that involves regular sessions with a health professional to review your diet, typically a **dietician**.

Dietician: A medical professional who deals with diet. Note that **dietician** is a legally protected term in the UK. In contrast, anyone can describe themselves as a **nutritionist**, which has no official meaning.

DNA: Deoxyribonucleic acid. Our genes.

Epigenetics: The study of how our genes express themselves. Our DNA is hard-coded: this is how nature made us. However, it is clear that nurture/environment can also affect our personalities. Think of our genes as the hardware, and how they express themselves as the software.

Exposure: The process of putting ourselves in uncomfortable situations to show our anxiety it is not as bad as we think. This should be done in a **graded** way, in which we break tasks down into manageable chunks.

GAD: See **generalised anxiety disorder**.

Generalised anxiety disorder: A type of anxiety diagnosis characterised by fears and worries that present themselves in everyday life, without specific triggers or situations.

GP: General practitioner. Your doctor.

Graded exposure: See **exposure**.

Hypnotic: A drug that induces sleep.

Insomnia: A chronic inability to sleep.

Interpersonal psychotherapy: A therapy that looks at the existing relationships in your life and the impact that they have on you.

Limbic system: A section of the brain made up of different systems used in memory, behaviour and emotion.

KCALs: See **kilocalories**.

Kilocalories: 1,000 calories. When people talk about calories, they are usually referring to **kilocalories**. For example, a typical adult may be advised to eat 2,000 kcals per day.

Mindfulness: The practice of bringing your attention to focus on the present moment. **Mindful-based therapy** has been developed to provide structures and systems to do this.

Muggle: Non-magic folk in J. K. Rowling's Harry Potter series. In this context, I use the term to refer to people without anxiety.

NAT: See negative automatic thought.

Naturalistic fallacy: The logical fallacy of assuming that because something is natural, it is good. Sunshine, vegetables and water are both natural and good. However, polio, famine and arsenic are all perfectly natural too, but not very good for you.

Negative automatic thought: A negative thought that you jump to without conscious intervention. For example, you think about learning something new, but your mind says "don't bother because you will fail".

Nonbenzodiazepines: A type of drug that has the same effects as **benzodiazepines**. It is chemically different and is therefore given a different label. For the patient, however, the experience is comparable.

OTC: Over-the-counter.

Oxytocin: A hormone, often referred to as the "love hormone". It is released during social bonding and plays a special role between intimate partners and mother and babies. In general, more oxytocin is good.

Placebo effect: The concept that thinking you are being treated, makes you better. For example, a doctor giving you medication which is just sugar pills. Because you think you are receiving treatment, you improve faster. It is a real, measurable effect. Injections work better than pills, and fake surgery works even better than that. It is mirrored by the ***nocebo effect*** which is where you expect a negative outcome, and are therefore more likely to get it. The ***placebo effect*** is the reason we need to split trials into two groups: a ***treatment group*** that gets the pill, and a ***control group*** that gets a placebo. Only be seeing a difference between these two groups can we actually know if the medication works, or other it is just a ***placebo effect***.

Psychotherapy: A broad term referring to mental health therapies. It includes cognitive-behavioural therapy and has a significant overlap with counselling.

REM sleep: Rapid eye movement sleep. This is a phase that usually occurs around 90 minutes after you fall asleep and is associated with dreaming.

SAD: See ***social anxiety disorder***.

Should statements: A form of negative automatic thoughts that use the word should. For example "I should be able to do this" or "I should be able to control my anxiety".

Social anxiety disorder: A type of anxiety characterised by a persistent and overwhelming fear of social situations.

Social phobia: Another term for ***social anxiety disorder***.

SSRI: Selective serotonin reuptake inhibitors. A type of antidepressant medication used to treat anxiety.

Tautology: A statement that says the same thing twice or is inherently true. For example "having fun is fun" or "what we will, will be".

The Lancet: A prestigious medical journal. ***The Lancet*** is currently ranked the second most authoritative medical journal, behind the ***New England Journal of Medicine***.

Therapist: Someone who delivers therapy.

Treatment group: See ***placebo effect***.

Z-drugs: See ***nonbenzodiazepines***.

Printed in Great Britain
by Amazon

16330103R00122